Handbook of

EEG
INTERPRETATION

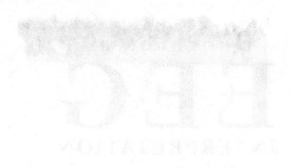

Handbook of
EEG
INTERPRETATION
Second Edition

Editor
William O. Tatum, IV, DO
Professor of Neurology
Mayo Clinic College of Medicine
Jacksonville, Florida

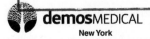

demosMEDICAL
New York

Visit our website at www.demosmedical.com

ISBN: **9781620700167**
e-book ISBN: **9781617051807**

Acquisitions Editor: Beth Barry
Compositor: diacriTech

Medicine is an ever-changing science. Research and clinical experience are continually expanding our knowledge, in particular our understanding of proper treatment and drug therapy. The authors, editors, and publisher have made every effort to ensure that all information in this book is in accordance with the state of knowledge at the time of production of the book. Nevertheless, the authors, editors, and publisher are not responsible for errors or omissions or for any consequences from application of the information in this book and make no warranty, expressed or implied, with respect to the contents of the publication. Every reader should examine carefully the package inserts accompanying each drug and should carefully check whether the dosage schedules mentioned therein or the contraindications stated by the manufacturer differ from the statements made in this book. Such examination is particularly important with drugs that are either rarely used or have been newly released on the market.

Library of Congress Cataloging-in-Publication Data
Handbook of EEG interpretation/editor, William O. Tatum, IV.—Second edition.
      p. ; cm.
  Includes bibliographical references and index.
  ISBN 978-1-62070-016-7—ISBN 978-1-61705-180-7 (e-book)
  I. Tatum, William O., IV, editor of compilation.
  [DNLM: 1. Electroencephalography—methods—Atlases. 2. Electroencephalography—methods—Handbooks. 3. Epilepsy—diagnosis—Atlases. 4. Epilepsy—diagnosis—Handbooks. 5. Monitoring, Physiologic—Atlases. 6. Monitoring, Physiologic—Handbooks. 7. Seizures—diagnosis—Atlases. 8. Seizures—diagnosis—Handbooks. WL 39]
  RC386.6.E43
  616.8'047547—dc23

                                                                          2013043217

Special discounts on bulk quantities of Demos Medical Publishing books are available to corporations, professional associations, pharmaceutical companies, health care organizations, and other qualifying groups. For details, please contact:

Special Sales Department
Demos Medical Publishing, LLC
11 West 42nd Street, 15th Floor
New York, NY 10036
Phone: 800-532-8663 or 212-683-0072
Fax: 212-941-7842
E-mail: specialsales@demosmedical.com

Printed in the United States of America by Edwards Brothers Malloy.
14 15 16 17 / 5 4 3 2 1

Contents

Contents

Preface

To properly preface this work, it must first be understood that the clinical interpretation of electroencephalography (EEG) is an art that involves an integral and necessary portion of neurology and of clinical neurophysiology. In any field of medicine, the best quality of care is proportional to the knowledge of the practitioner. In the case of EEG, this knowledge is a function of experience and, for most, experience is a function of exposure. Historically, neophyte electroencephalographers have acquired their fund of knowledge during their training programs. Learning from those who are more senior in experience and knowledge within the field of EEG provides the template that demands ongoing supplementation of their skill. While much of EEG education occurs during their training, learning begins often outside the classroom when real life experiences force commitment from actual patient experiences. EEG "at the bedside" is where critical learning begins—where decisions are made based upon dynamic information that at times is critical to discern the correct choice of treatment.

This second edition of the "Handbook" gained momentum following the widespread success of the first edition. New chapters, including ICU EEG, Status Epilepticus, and Pediatric EEG, are now included in this version to reflect the advances in applications that are surfacing. The chapters outlined in this book are intended to be used as a supplement to clinical experience and continued education to ensure proper use of EEG results. The "bottom line" is provided within each chapter to help readers address the principal challenges involved with EEG interpretation focused on individual topics. Like the original, the second edition is intended to provide an appreciation of the essentials of EEG interpretation and improve one's acumen in EEG use in clinical neurophysiology. The expanded focus reflects the growth within the field of neurophysiology, which has evolved to include new disciplines and techniques.

Our hope in providing quick and easy access to key topics in EEG is that patients will ultimately receive better care. Correctly delineating normal and abnormal EEG patterns represents a hugely important skill set for clinicians. Recognizing epileptiform abnormalities and identifying ictal EEG patterns in and outside special care units for children and adults is the essence of EEG. The importance of this technology in defining chronic treatment where it serves as the ideal (and in some cases the singular) study for evaluating patients with seizures cannot be understated. Patterns of special significance may be seen in patients with encephalopathy manifest as stupor and coma overlapping with those patients that are experiencing status epilepticus. Chapters on sleep and neurointensive intraoperative monitoring add useful information to complete the handbook for clinicians that would benefit from quick and easy pattern recognition.

There are many excellent comprehensive clinical works that have served to advance our knowledge of EEG. We have tried instead to condense the fundamental knowledge and contain it within a portable handbook, to provide the reader with a "bullet" of information complete with a graphic representation of the principal features in EEG that is operational during crucial bedside interpretation of a patient's "brainwaves." We have written *Handbook of EEG Interpretation* to fit into the lab coat pockets of *all* health care professionals who need or desire access to quick, reliable EEG information, regardless of specialty or level of training. Whether one is young or old; new or learned; for those interested in the field of EEG, we hope you enjoy the study design of the handbook. EEG represents a "window to the brain" to augment the clinical acumen of the practitioner. We trust that the second edition of this book will again provide a portable service for our colleagues and our patients. As clinical applications for this unique technology multiply, we can anticipate that EEG will continue to find new roles that benefit from its use within the great field of clinical neurophysiology.

William O. Tatum, IV, DO

Contributors

Selim R. Benbadis, MD
Director, Comprehensive Epilepsy Program
Tampa General Hospital;
Professor, Departments of Neurology and Neurosurgery
University of South Florida
Tampa, Florida

Frank W. Drislane, MD
Director, Inpatient Epilepsy and Consultative Services
Beth Israel Deaconess Medical Center;
Professor, Department of Neurology
Harvard Medical School
Boston, Massachusetts

Nicolas Gaspard, MD, PhD
Postdoctoral Research Associate
Department of Neurology
Comprehensive Epilepsy Center and Computational Neurophysiology Lab
Yale University School of Medicine
New Haven, Connecticut

Lawrence J. Hirsch, MD
Chief, Division of Epilepsy/EEG
Yale Comprehensive Epilepsy Center;
Professor, Department of Neurology
Yale University School of Medicine
New Haven, Connecticut

Aatif M. Husain, MD
Professor, Department of Neurology
Duke University Medical Center;
Director, Neurodiagnostic Center
Veterans Affairs Medical Center
Durham, North Carolina

Peter W. Kaplan, MB, FRCP
Professor, Department of Neurology
Johns Hopkins Bayview Medical Center
Baltimore, Maryland

Douglas R. Nordli, Jr, MD
Lorna S. and James P. Landgon Chair of Pediatric Epilepsy
Ann & Robert H. Lurie Children's Hospital of Chicago;
Professor of Pediatrics
Northwestern University Feinberg School of Medicine
Chicago, Illinois

William O. Tatum, IV, DO
Professor of Neurology
Mayo Clinic College of Medicine
Jacksonville, Florida

Will Underwood, RPSGT
Lab Manager
University of North Carolina Hospital Sleep Center
Chapel Hill, North Carolina

Bradley V. Vaughn, MD
Professor, Departments of Neurology, Biomedical Engineering, and Allied Health
University of North Carolina School of Medicine
Chapel Hill, North Carolina

1

Normal EEG

William O. Tatum, IV

The value of understanding the normal electroencephalogram (EEG) lies in developing the foundation to identify an abnormality with clinical relevance. Knowledge of normal waveform variations, variants of normal or uncertain significance, and variability and fluctuation of the normal EEG throughout the lifecycle are therefore essential to provide an accurate clinical interpretation. When abnormality is in doubt, a conservative impression of "normal" is recommended to avoid adversely influencing a clinical treatment which may be unnecessary.

The EEG is a unique and valuable measure of the brain's electrical function. It is a graphic display of a difference in voltages from two sites of brain function recorded over time. Electroencephalography (EEG) involves the study of recording these electrical signals that are generated by the brain. Extracranial scalp-based EEG provides a broad survey of the electrocerebral activity throughout both hemispheres of the brain. Intracranial EEG provides a direct brain recording obtained through surgically implanted electrodes. These electrode recordings target specific regions in the brain. Information about diffuse or focal cerebral dysfunction, the presence of interictal epileptiform discharges (IEDs), and periodic and ictal EEG patterns can be seen that drastically impact the approach to patient management. For the successful interpretation of an abnormal EEG one must first understand the criteria necessary to define normal patterns. While a normal EEG does not exclude a clinical diagnosis (e.g., epilepsy), an abnormal finding on EEG may be diagnostic of a particular diagnosis (e.g., nonconvulsive status epilepticus), indicate the process for cerebral dysfunction (e.g., focal or generalized slowing), or reveal features on the EEG that are irrelevant to the reason that the study was performed (e.g., in headache). Even a normal EEG may provide extremely useful information and function as a "window" to the brain to define the clinical situation (e.g., psychogenic unresponsiveness). It is the clinical application of the EEG findings that represents its principal importance and directs its utility to improve patient outcomes.

BASIC PHYSIOLOGY OF CEREBRAL POTENTIALS

The origin of cerebral potentials is based upon the intrinsic electro-physiological properties of the nervous system. Identifying the generator source(s) and electrical field(s) of propagation are the basis for recognizing electrographic patterns that underly the expression of the "brain waves" as normal or abnormal. Most routine EEGs recorded at the surface of the scalp represent pooled electrical activity generated by large numbers of neurons.

Electrical signals are created when electrical charges move within the central nervous system. Neural function is normally maintained by *ionic gradients* established by neuronal membranes. Sufficient duration and length of small amounts (in microvolts) of electrical currents of cerebral activity are required to be amplified and displayed for interpretation. A *resting (diffusion) membrane potential* normally exists through the efflux of positive-charged (potassium) ions maintaining an *electrochemical equilibrium* of –75 mV. With *depolarization*, an influx of positive-charged (sodium) ions that exceeds the normal electrochemical resting state occurs. Channel opening within the lipid bilayer is via a voltage-dependent mechanism, and closure is time dependent. Conduction to adjacent portions of the nerve cell membranes results in an action potential when the depolarization threshold is exceeded. However, it is the *synaptic potentials* that are the most important source of the extracellular current flow that produces cerebral potentials that are seen after amplification in the EEG. *Excitatory postsynaptic potentials* (EPSPs) flow inwardly (extracellular to intracellular) to other parts of the cell *(sinks)* via sodium or calcium ions. *Inhibitory postsynaptic potentials* (IPSPs) flow outwardly (intracellular to extracellular) in the opposite direction *(source)*, and involve chloride or potassium ions. These summed potentials are longer in duration than action potentials and are responsible for most of the EEG waveforms. The brainstem and thalamus serve as subcortical generators to synchronize populations of neocortical neurons in both normal (e.g., sleep elements) and in abnormal situations (e.g., generalized spike-and-wave complexes). *Volume conduction* characterizes the process of current flow from the brain generator and recording electrode. The *pyramidal cells* are the major contributor of the synaptic potentials that make up EEG (Figure 1.1A).

These neurons are arranged in a perpendicular orientation to the cortical surface from *layers III, IV,* and *VI.* Volumes large enough to allow measurement at the surface of the scalp require greater than 10 cm^2 for most IEDs to appear on the scalp EEG because of the attenuating properties incurred by the skull. All generators have both a positive and negative pole that functions as a *dipole* (Figure 1.1B). The EEG displays the continuous and changing voltage fields varying with different locations on the scalp over time.

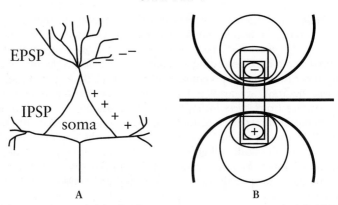

FIGURE 1.1. (A) A pyramidal cell with excitatory postsynaptic potentials and inhibitory postsynaptic potentials. (B) Dipole depicting a field of charge separation. EPSP = excitatory postsynaptic potentials; IPSP = inhibitory postsynaptic potentials.

Scalp EEG recording displays the difference in electrical potentials between two different sites on the head overlying cerebral cortex that is closest to the recording electrode. During routine use, electrical potentials are acquired indirectly from the scalp surface and incorporate waveform analyses of frequency, voltage, morphology, and topography. However, most of the human cortex is buried deep beneath the scalp surface, and additionally represents a two-dimensional projection of a three-dimensional source, presenting a problem for generator localization in scalp EEG. Furthermore, the waveforms that are recorded from the scalp represent *pooled synchronous activity* from large populations of neurons that create the cortical potentials and may not represent small interictal or ictal sources.

Initial one-channel EEG recordings in the late 1920s have evolved to sophisticated digital-based computerized recording devices. From the patient scalp, EEG electrodes conduct electrical potentials to an *electrode box* (jackbox). Thereafter, a montage selector permits EEG signals to pass through amplifiers before filtering and other parameter controls regulate the signal output. Data display follows acquisition and processing and has a wide variety of data presentation for EEG interpretation. Electrode placement has been standardized by the international 10-20 system that uses anatomical landmarks on the skull. These sites are then subdivided by intervals of 10% to 20% and designate the site where an electrode will be placed. A minimum of 21 electrodes are recommended for clinical study, although digital EEG now has the capability for a much greater number. During infant EEG recordings, fewer electrodes are used depending upon age and head size. The modified combinatorial electrode system uses electrode placement with more closely spaced electrodes in a 10-10 system of scalp EEG recording (Figure 1.2). The designations; Fp (frontopolar), F (frontal), T (temporal), O (occipital), C (central), and P (parietal) are utilized in the 10-20 system. Subsequently, numbers combined following the letters for location reflect either the left (odd numbers) or right (even numbers) hemisphere of electrode placement. The "z" designation reflects midline placement (e.g., Cz = central midline). In the 10-10 system, lower numbers in their positions reflect locations closer to the midline, and T3/T4 become T7/T8, while T5/T6 become P7/P8. Electrode impedances should be maintained between 100 and 5000 ohms. Special electrodes may also be added such as sphenoidal, true temporal, or frontotemporal electrodes. Most are employed for the purpose of delineating temporal localization. True temporal electrodes (designated T1 and T2) are placed to help distinguish anterior temporal or posterior inferior frontal location not delineated by the F7 or F8 positions. Combining the 10-20 system with electrodes from the 10-10 system may be most practical for routine clinical use as additional electrodes become desired. Colloidion is a compound used to secure electrodes during prolonged recording techniques such as during video-EEG or ambulatory monitoring. Paste used for routine recordings is more temporary. Subdermal electrodes are used when other recording techniques are not feasible such as in the OR and ICU.

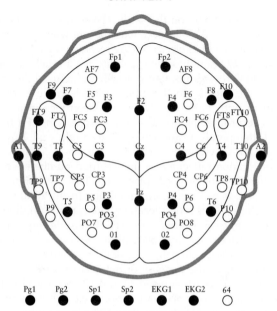

FIGURE 1.2. Electrode placements systems use either a 10-20 system (black circles) or modified combinatorial system with 10-10 electrode placement (black circles + white circles).

Other added electrodes may include electrocardiogram (EKG) (recommended with every EEG), eye movement monitors, electromyogram (EMG), and extracerebral electrodes to aid in artifact differentiation, or with sleep staging in the case of eye lead monitors. Respiratory monitors may also be important if respiratory problems are identified.

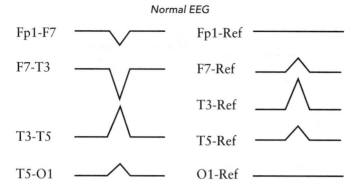

FIGURE 1.3. (A) A bipolar montage demonstrates phase reversals and (B) a referential montage demonstrates absolute voltage. In this example T3 is the site of maximal electronegativity.

The electrical "map" that is developed from the spatial array of recording electrodes used is the montage. Several montages are used throughout a 20- to 30-minute routine EEG recording. Every routine EEG should include at least one montage using a longitudinal bipolar, reference, and traverse bipolar montage (Figures 1.3 and 1.4). A reference montage uses an active electrode site as the initial input, and then at least one "neutral" electrode to depict absolute voltage through amplitude measurement that is commensurate with the area of maximal electronegativity or postivity (Figure 1.3B). A midline reference electrode (e.g., Pz), may be useful for lateralizing temporal recordings. However, two references (e.g., ipsilateral ear reference) may be useful for more generalized discharges. Even multiple "averaged" sites of reference (or Laplacian montages for very focal recordings) may be useful for localized discharges. Bipolar montages may be arranged in many different spatial formats including longitudinally, transverse fashion, or in a circumferential pattern. The longitudinal bipolar (also called "double banana") is frequently represented throughout this text. An anterior to posterior temporal and central connecting chain of electrodes arranged left alternating with right-sided placement is a typical array. Bipolar montages compare active electrodes sites adjacent to each other and signify absolute electrographic sites of maximal negativity (or positivity) by phase reversals (Figure 1.3A).

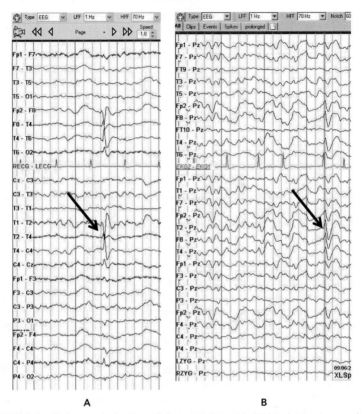

FIGURE 1.4. Right temporal spike and slow-wave (arrow) in (A) bipolar montage and (B) referential montage. Note the maximal electronegativity occurs at T2.

EEG	Electrode 1	Electrode 2
Negative	Up	Down
Positive	Down	Up

FIGURE 1.5. The rule governing polarity and convention is relative to "pen" deflection. When input 1 is negative the deflection is up.

By convention, when the voltage difference between electrode 1 is more negative than electrode 2, deflection of the waveform is *up*. Recordings are usually performed with a visual display of 30 mm/sec (slower with sleep studies), amplifier sensitivities of 7 µV/mm, and filter settings have routinely consisted of 1 to 70 Hz. Reducing the low filter setting promotes slower frequency representation, while reducing high filter settings reduces the high frequencies. A narrow band reduction is possible using a notched filter setting to limit 60-Hz interference (50-Hz in the UK). Proprietary software offers seizure and spike detection capabilities for digital EEG systems that are commercially available for both routine and prolonged EEG monitoring. This section will encompass patterns of cerebral and extracerebral origin, as well as patterns of uncertain significance to illustrate the range of normal EEGs encountered in clinical practice.

EXTRACEREBRAL ARTIFACTS

Recording electrical activity from the brain is subject to noncerebral activity referred to as "interference." Various generators of nonphysiological and physiological artifacts may deceive the interpreter to believe that the apparent sources are abnormal or epileptiform. When in doubt, it is incumbent upon the EEG interpreter to assume that the source is an artifact until proven otherwise.

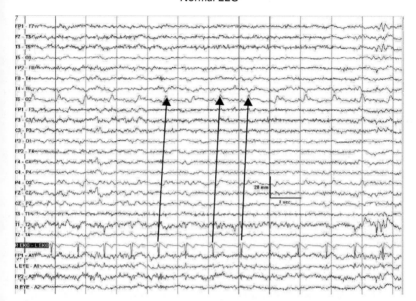

FIGURE 1.6. Pulse artifact can mimic periodic lateralized discharges in this example noted at the T6 derivation. Note the 1:1 relationship to the EKG (arrows) and the electrical field that is limited to a single electrode present with pulse artifact.

The EKG should be monitored during EEG to provide information about the relationship between the heart and the brain. The QRS complex of the EEG represents the largest deflection and often confers artifact. An EKG artifact may appear simultaneously with prominent QRS complexes seen in several channels. Ballistocardiographic potentials reveal a movement artifact that is time locked to the EKG. In the example above, pulse artifact is seen that is usually present in a single channel manifest as a periodic slow wave. It occurs when an electrode is in a position near an artery that detects pulsation of blood flow initiated by the heartbeat. There is, therefore, a discrete time-locked 1:1 relationship between the heart rate and the periodic potential that is produced by the surge of arterial blood flow to generate the corresponding artifact on the EEG.

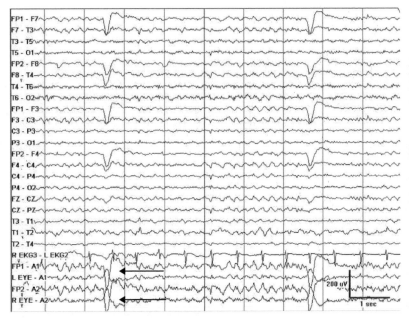

FIGURE 1.7. Eye movement monitors demonstrate the *in-phase* cerebral origin of the diffusely slow background activity in an awake patient. Note the *out-of-phase* deflection or phase-reversing (arrows) that is present in FP1-A1/FP2-A2 and L EYE-A1/R EYE-A2 during the vertical eye blink artifact in seconds 3 and 8.

An eye blink artifact seen in the EEG (see above) is generated by the electrical potential produced by vertical movement of the eye. Normally, the eye functions as an electrical dipole with a relative positivity of the cornea compared to the retina. The potential created is a DC potential of higher amplitude (mV) than the amplitude produced by the brain (µV). The artifact is produced in the electrodes around the eye (FP1/2) during vertical eye movements. With an eye blink, the cornea rolls up with resultant positivity in the FP1/2 electrodes relative to the F3/4 electrodes and creates a downward deflection during the normal Bell's phenomenon. Electrodes recording above and below the eye will help to distinguish the brain as the "generator" (same polarity is every channel) from an artifact (opposite polarity in electrode sites above and below the eye).

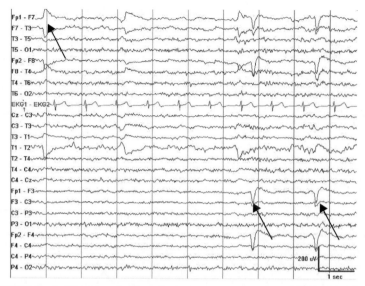

FIGURE 1.8. Artifact generated from three eye movements composed of horizontal eye movements (first arrow looking left) followed by two vertical eye blinks (second and third arrows).

The presence of vertical eye blink artifact helps define the state of the patient as being awake. During drowsiness, slow rolling (lateral) eye movements are similarly helpful. Lateral eye movements are usually easily recognized because they create phase reversals in the anterior temporal derivations that are of opposite polarity on opposite sides of the scalp EEG. When the eyes move to the left, yielding a positive phase reversal in F7 due to the cornea polarity, the homologous F8 electrode site demonstrates a negative phase reversal that is generated by the retina. Note the two lateral eye movements at the end of second 1 and during second 4 in Figure 1.8. The positive phase reversals noted at the F8 derivation is due to the proximity of the cornea. The homologous F7 electrode site is negative due to the conjugate effect from the retina.

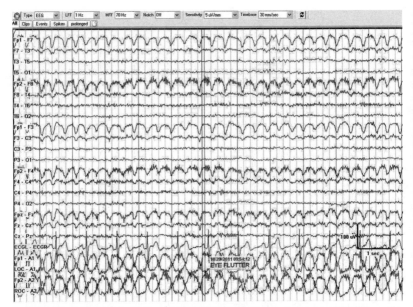

FIGURE 1.9. Continuous vertical eye flutter artifact identified with infraorbital electrodes differentiating artifact from frontal intermittent rhythmic delta activity. Note the out-of-phase eye movement monitors in the lower four channels.

Detecting eye movements may be accomplished using a single channel connecting the right upper lateral eyebrow and the left lower lateral eyebrow. However, because vertical eye movements may be confused with frontal slowing or in some cases frontal sharp waves, bilateral infraorbital electrodes (referred to the ipsilateral ear as a reference) may better represent the eye as an electrical dipole and demonstrate phase reversals that are out-of-phase with cerebral activity when the waveforms are due to eye movements (see above). Eye movement monitors may be added during the recording if difficulty differentiating cerebral function from extracerebral origin becomes desirable, though our center uses them during routine recordings.

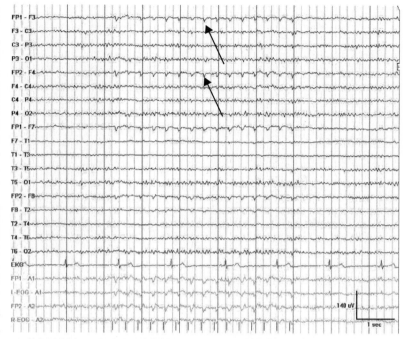

FIGURE 1.10. The electroretinogram (arrows) seen at the FP1/2 electrodes less than 50 msec after the flash associated with intermittent photic stimulation.

The electroretinogram (ERG) is a normal response of the retina to photic stimulation. The amplitude is usually low voltage and appears in the anterior head regions. Normally an A and B wave occurs during photic flash as an evoked potential recording. However, the ERG can also be seen on the EEG and become confused with abnormal frontal sharp waves. To distinguish the ERG from the photoelectric effect, covering the electrodes with a cloth will demonstrate the persistence of the potentials in the ERG. Additionally, using high rates of IPSP will fatigue the retinal response.

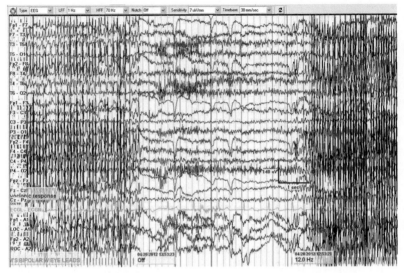

FIGURE 1.11. A reproducible photomyoclonic response during intermittent photic stimulation. The myogenic "polyspikes" are due to artifact that is maximal in the fronto-polar EEG channels created by contraction of the frontalis muscles.

The photomyoclonic response is an extracerebral response obtained from the frontalis muscles of the scalp. Contraction of the anterior muscles of the scalp produces EMG artifact that vary from single to sustained myogenic potentials. The contractions are time locked to the frequency of intermittent photic stimulation and begin and cease commensurate with each flash, although there is often a brief delay between the flash and the myogenic potentials that appear. The principal confusion that may result is when one mistakenly identifies a normal photomyoclonic response with an abnormal photoparoxysmal response (see above).

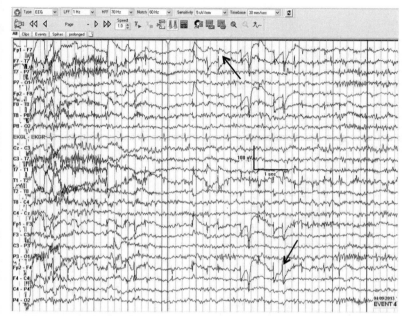

FIGURE 1.12. Prominent lateral rectus spikes (arrows) during rapid eye movements. Myogenic spikes occur due to contraction of the lateral recti and may be confused with pathological epileptiform discharges.

Patients with rapid eye movements may demonstrate myogenic potentials from the lateral rectus muscles that may appear epileptiform in appearance. Each rapid eye movement is associated with a positive potential represented by a phase reversal upon eye deviation toward the side of the lateral rectus that is contracting. These can be present during the awake state (Figure 1.12) or during REM sleep.

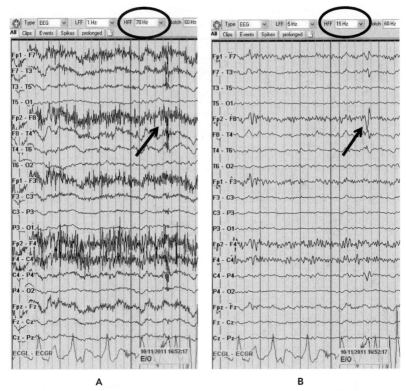

FIGURE 1.13. (A) Bitemporal myogenic artifact during second 4 produced by the temporalis musculature. (B) Note the effect of over-filtering creating an apparent sharp wave (arrow). High frequency filters are identified by the ovals.

A myogenic (muscle) artifact consists of brief potentials that may occur individually or become continuous, obscuring underlying EEG. EMG activity that is produced during a seizure, individual muscle contraction, or with movement is due to increased muscle tone. This artifact is most prominent in individuals who are tense during the EEG and is maximal in the temporal or frontopolar derivations of the EEG over the site of the temporalis and frontalis muscles. Myogenic potentials are composed of high-frequency activity that is much briefer than the greater than 20-msec potentials encountered with IEDs unless inappropriate filter settings are applied (Figure 1.13). In addition, an aftergoing slow wave is absent. Having the individual relax their jaw muscles or capturing sleep will lead to waning or elimination of myogenic artifact.

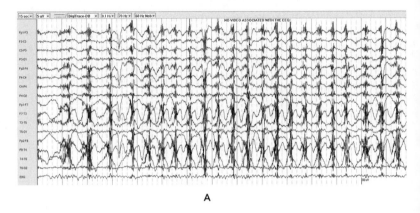

A

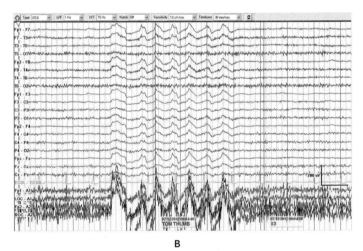

B

FIGURE 1.14. (A) Chewing artifact seen at regular 1 sec intervals on ambulatory EEG. Note the myogenic artifact is maximal in the bitemporal regions because the temporalis muscle is a principal site of mastication. (B) Glossokinetic artifact mimicking frontal intermittent rhythmic delta activity. Note the "in-phase" deflections of the eye movement monitors due to the generator arising inferior to the eye.

(Continued)

Regular bursts of myogenic potentials are seen during chewing. These high-voltage temporal predominant bursts are due to contraction of the muscles associated with mastication. Associated "slow" potentials during chewing reflect associated swallowing movements created by the tongue. The tongue, like the eye, acts as a dipole with the tip of the tongue being positive relative to the root. The chewing produces myogenic "polyspike" artifact created by the temporalis muscles and may be accompanied thereafter by the slower glossokinetic movements of the tongue to produce confusion with IEDs, especially if video is absent to provide a behavioral correlation.

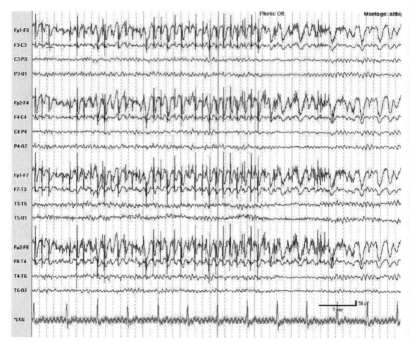

FIGURE 1.15. A photomyoclonic response during intermittent photic stimulation. Notice the apparent spike-and-wave pattern due to artifact in the frontopolar channels produced by the frontalis musculature created in the frontopolar channels.

Superimposition of background frequencies can be deceiving when normal, physiological, and artifact are combined. Identifying normal morphologies within the background and comparing the frequencies of one or a series of suspicious waveforms may help separate a normal from an abnormal pattern. In the above example, combined artifacts (eye flutter and muscle artifact) create the appearance of a photoparoxysmal response during intermittent photic stimulation. The appearance superficially could be a pitfall to novice interpreters.

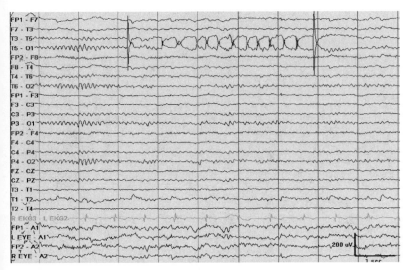

FIGURE 1.16A. A single electrode artifact evident at T5.

Potentials that are confined to a single electrode derivation are highly suspicious for a single (or common electrode in average/linked montages) electrode artifact. Identifying a single electrode artifact should prompt a technologist to check the impedance and resecure the electrode scalp-electrolyte interface, change the electrode if a persistent artifact remains, and/or move the electrode to an alternate channel to determine if the artifact in the channel remains signifying the channel/jackbox itself is defective.

(Continued)

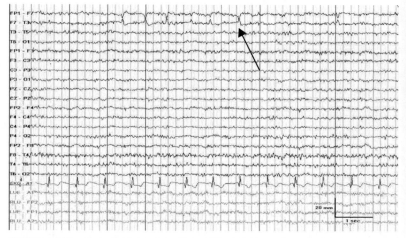

FIGURE 1.16B. A single electrode artifact at F7 mimicking a sharp wave (arrow).

Bizarre morphologies may occur and are usually recognizable. Occasionally, a single electrode artifact may mimic sharp waves (see above). Despite the "sharp wave" morphological appearance, any waveform isolated to a single channel of EEG should be interpreted as artifact until proven otherwise.

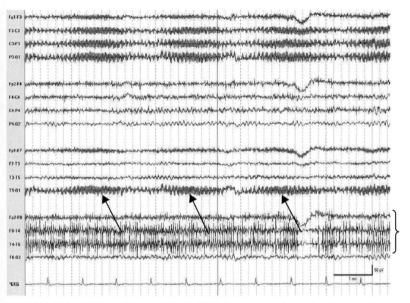

FIGURE 1.17A. 60-Hz artifact noted in the EEG. Note the regular cycling (arrows) of the 60 Hz frequencies as opposed to the continuous fast frequencies of muscle artifact (brackets).

A 60-cycle artifact is a function of the circuitry of the amplifiers and common mode rejection when electrode impedances are unequal. The frequency of an electrical line is represented in the EEG usually when poor electrode impedances produce a mismatch. This artifact should prompt a search for electrodes with an impedance of greater than 5000 ohm when a single electrode is involved, as well as ensuring that ground loops and double grounds do not put the patient at a safety risk when a generalized 60-cycle artifact is found, as in the above example.

(Continued)

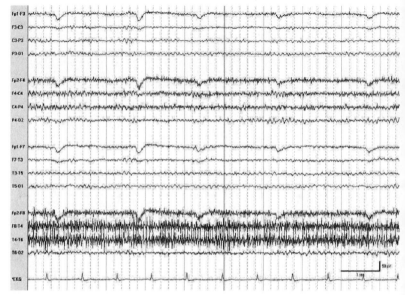

FIGURE 1.17B. Resolution of the 60-Hz artifact occurs following the application of a notched filter.

After the application of the 60-Hz notched filter, note the elimination of the artifact that was seen on page 25 permitting interpretation of an interpretable EEG. However, notice the persistent right temporal myogenic artifact in the example above has remained due to the narrow range of the notched frequency filtration that occurs at 60 Hz leaving other frequencies (artifactual or otherwise) unfiltered.

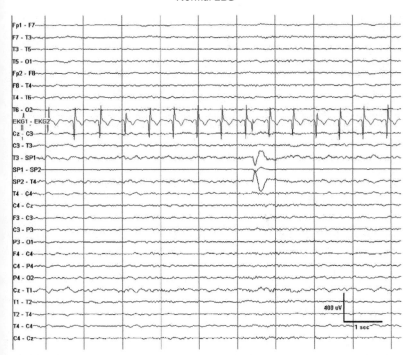

FIGURE 1.18. Artifact in the sphenoidal electrodes due to open channels in the jackbox that appears as a temporal sharp wave. Note the limited electrophysiological field that is apparent.

Some electrode artifacts are difficult to recognize. In the above example, the sphenoidal derivations were not functional and created an electrode artifact that closely mimicked a temporal sharp wave. Note the lack of a believable cerebral field and the absence of any deflection in the true temporal and lateral temporal derivations despite the high amplitude represented by the scale legend in the bottom right-hand corner.

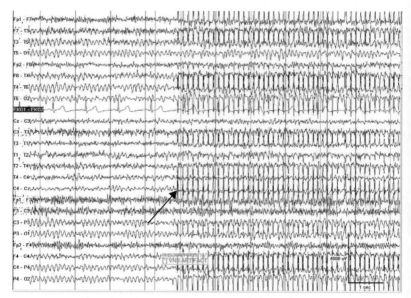

FIGURE 1.19. Vagus nerve stimulation (VNS) artifact on the right (arrow) recorded during active stimulation during continuous video-EEG monitoring.

An electrical artifact occurs when electronic circuits that may be caused by surgically implanted devices (such as pacemakers or vagus nerve stimulation [VNS]) produce undesirable signals internally that contaminate the EEG or EKG recording. In this way, the patient or unshielded electrodes act as an antenna and produce extracerebral sources of artifact similar to the way nearby power lines may create external 60-Hz interference by the induction of magnetic fields created from nearby current flow. It is the current flow that results in electrode depolarization, is amplified by the amplifiers, and creates the resultant "noise."

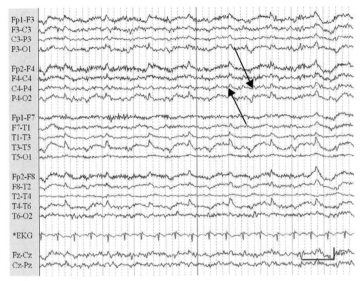

FIGURE 1.20. A mechanical artifact induced by continuous positive airway pressure (CPAP) in a comatose patient in the intensive care unit (ICU). Note the alternating polarity (arrows) of the mechanical artifact superimposed on a low voltage background.

A variety of artifacts can be seen in the intensive care unit (ICU), critical care unit (CCU), or clinical specialty unit (CSU) produced by mechanical or instrumental sources. Electrical induced "noise" can be more evident for routine mechanical function at high gain (low sensitivity) settings. Alternating movement generated by a respirator is noted in the above example using high sensitivities of 3 µV/mm in a patient who is intubated and mechanically ventilated with continuous positive airway pressure (CPAP).

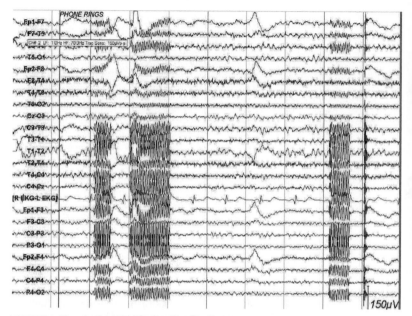

FIGURE 1.21. A telephone ring artifact produced by an incoming call that occurred during in-patient long-term video-EEG monitoring.

Environmental artifacts may be quite elusive. They may often not be readily identifiable or correctable within the confines of a "hostile" environment when performing EEG in the ICU or CCU. Some of these artifacts may be generated by high frequencies produced by nearby electrical machinery not directly connected to the patient. Equipment such as blood warmers, bovies, and electrical beds in the operating room (OR) may be challenging to locate the source of the artifact. By unplugging or moving equipment away from the recording electrode, redirecting electrical current flow may eliminate the artifact from the EEG. Telephone lines (see above) may interfere with EEG and produce an artifact typically in all the channels during recording.

The application of routine EEG provides information about generators emanating from a three-dimensional sphere with regard to location, distribution, waveform frequency, polarity, and morphology. The state of wakefulness and age are critical features for accurate interpretation of the normal EEG.

NORMAL WAVEFORMS

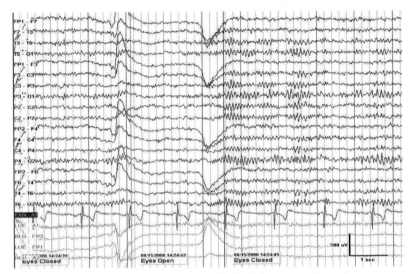

FIGURE 1.22. A normal 10-Hz alpha rhythm "blocked" by eye opening and returning on eye closure. Note the faster frequency immediately on eye closure ("alpha squeak").

The alpha rhythm is the starting point to analyze clinical EEG. In the normal EEG, a posterior dominant rhythm is represented bilaterally over the posterior head regions and lies within the 8- to 13-Hz bandwidth (*alpha frequency*). When this rhythm is attenuated with eye opening, it is referred to as the *alpha rhythm*. During normal development, an 8-Hz alpha frequency appears by 3 years of age. The alpha rhythm remains stable between 8 and 13 Hz and remains stable throughout normal aging into the later years of life. In approximately 25% of normal adults, the alpha rhythm is poorly visualized, and in less than 10%, voltages of less than 15 μV may be seen. The alpha rhythm is distributed maximally in the occipital regions, and shifts anteriorly during drowsiness. Voltage asymmetries of greater than 50% should be regarded as abnormal, especially when the left side is greater than the right. It is best observed during relaxed wakefulness, and has a side to side difference of less than 1 Hz. Unilateral failure of the alpha rhythm to attenuate reflects an ipsilateral abnormality *(Bancaud's phenomenon)*. Normally, alpha frequencies may transiently increase immediately after eye closure *(alpha squeak)*. Alpha variants include forms that are one-half (slow alpha) or two times (fast alpha) the frequency with similar distribution and reactivity. Alpha variants may have a notched appearance. *Paradoxical alpha* occurs when alertness results in the presence of alpha, and drowsiness does not.

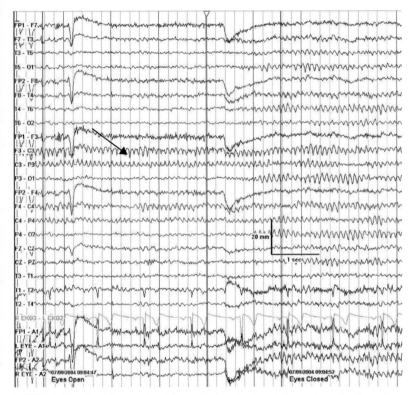

FIGURE 1.23. Note the prominent left central mu rhythm during eye opening (arrow) that persists despite "blocking" of the alpha rhythm.

The mu rhythm is a centrally located arciform alpha frequency (usually 8 to 10 Hz) that represents the sensorimotor cortex at rest (Figure 1.23). While it resembles the alpha rhythm, it does not block with eye opening, but instead with contralateral movement of an extremity. It may be seen only on one side, and may be quite asymmetrical and asynchronous, despite the notable absence of an underlying structural lesion. The mu rhythm may slow with advancing age, and is usually of lower amplitude than the existent alpha rhythm. When persistent, unreactive, and associated with focal slowing, mu-like frequencies are abnormal.

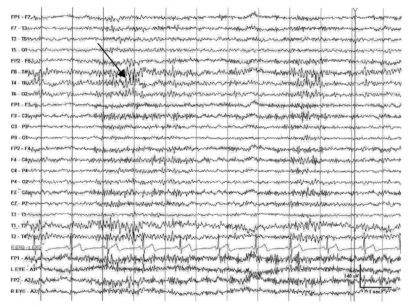

FIGURE 1.24. Breach rhythm in the right temporal region (maximal at T4) following craniotomy for temporal lobectomy (arrow).

Beta rhythms are frequencies that are higher than 13 Hz. They are commonly seen in the routine normal EEG and typically observed within the 18- to 25-Hz bandwidth with a voltage of less than 20 μV. Voltages beyond 25 μV in amplitude are abnormal. Benzodiazepines, barbiturates, and chloral hydrate are potent generalized beta activators of "fast activity" that is often greater than 50 μV for greater than 50% of the waking tracing within the 14- to 16-Hz bandwidth. Beta activity normally increases during drowsiness, light sleep, and with mental activation. Persistently reduced voltages of greater than 50% suggest a cortical gray matter abnormality within the hemisphere having the lower amplitude; however, lesser asymmetries may simply reflect normal skull asymmetries. A skull defect may produce a *breach rhythm* with focal, asymmetrical, higher amplitudes (this relative increase may be more than three times) beta activity without the skull to attenuate the faster frequencies. It is a normal finding expected within the conditions of the recording unless it is associated with spikes or focal slowing.

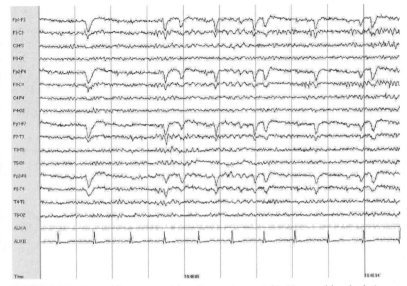

FIGURE 1.25. Normal frontocentral theta is seen in an awake 18-year-old male during concentration.

Theta rhythms are composed of 4- to 7-Hz frequencies of varying amplitude and morphologies. Approximately one-third of normal young adults may show intermittent 6- to 7-Hz theta rhythms of less than 15 µV that is maximal in the frontal or frontocentral head regions during wakefulness. The appearance of frontal theta can be facilitated by emotions, focused concentration, and during mental tasks. Theta activity is normally enhanced by hyperventilation, drowsiness, and sleep. Intermittent 4- to 5-Hz activity bitemporally, or even with a lateralized predominance (usually left greater than right), may occur in about one-third of the asymptomatic elderly and is not abnormal.

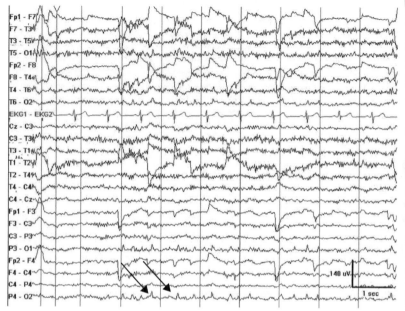

FIGURE 1.26. Biooccipital lambda waves in a 28-year-old patient with dizziness (arrows). Notice the frequent "scanning" eye movement artifact in the F7 and T8 derivations.

Lambda waves have been initially described as surface positive sharply contoured theta waves appearing bilaterally in the occipital region. These potentials have a duration of 160 to 250 msec, and may at times be quite sharply contoured, asymmetrical, with higher amplitudes than the resting posterior dominant rhythm. When they occur asymmetrically, there may be confusion with IEDs, and potentially lead to the misinterpretation of the EEG. They are best observed in young adults when seen, although they are more frequently found in children. Lambda waves are best elicited when the patient visually scans a textured or complex picture with fast saccadic eye movements. Placing a white sheet of paper in front of the individual will eliminate the visual input that is essential for their genesis.

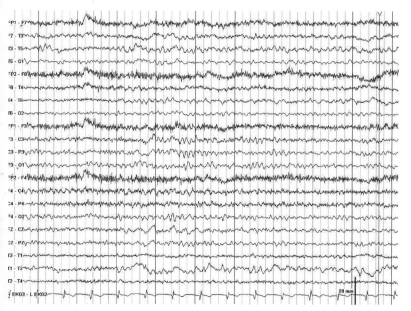

FIGURE 1.27. Intermittent left mid-temporal delta during transition to drowsiness in a normal 84-year-old patient evaluated for syncope.

Delta rhythms are frequencies consisting of less than 4-Hz activity that comprises less than 10% of the normal waking EEG by age 10. In the waking states, delta can be considered a normal finding in the very young and in the elderly. The normal elderly may have rare irregular delta complexes in the temporal regions. It is similar to temporal theta in the distribution, often left greater than right temporal head regions, but normally is present for less than 1% of the recording. Some delta is normal in people older than 60 years, at the onset of drowsiness, in response to hyperventilation, and during N3 sleep. Excessive generalized delta is abnormal and indicates an encephalopathy that is etiology nonspecific. Focal arrhythmic delta usually indicates a structural lesion involving the white matter of the ipsilateral hemisphere, especially when it is continuous and unreactive.

NORMAL SLEEP ARCHITECTURE

Interpreting sleep is an essential part of the normal EEG. A more detailed description is represented in Chapter 7. In this section we will concentrate on normal sleep architecture that may be seen in the routine scalp EEG. When wakefulness or stage W progresses to stage N1 sleep, the presence of vertex waves, typically appearing as 200-msec diphasic sharp transients with maximal negativity at the vertex (Cz) electrode are seen and may persist to N3 sleep. V-waves are bilateral, synchronous, and symmetrical, and may be induced by auditory stimuli. Vertex waves can appear spiky (especially in children) but should normally never be consistently lateralized. Other features include attenuation of the alpha rhythm, greater frontal prominence of beta, slow rolling eye movements, and vertex sharp transients. In addition, positive occipital sharp transients (POSTs) are another feature signifying stage N1 sleep (Figure 1.28). These are surface positive, bisynchronous physiological sharp waves with voltage asymmetries that may occur over the occipital regions as single complexes or in repetitive bursts that may be present in both stages N1 and N2 sleep.

(*Continued*)

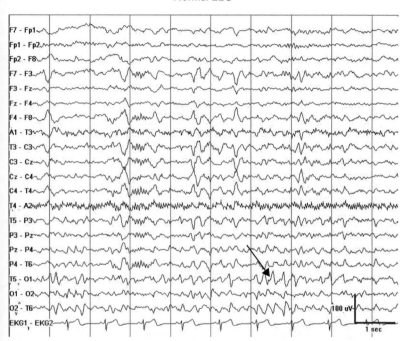

FIGURE 1.28. Positive occipital sharp transients (POSTs) appear in the lower three channels in a transverse bipolar circle montage demonstrating positive polarity in the occipital region during sleep (arrow). Notice the surface negative vertex waves are maximal at Cz, Fz, and Pz identified by the negative phase reversal.

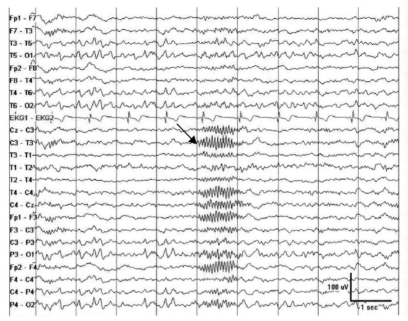

FIGURE 1.29. Stage N2 sleep with prominent sleep spindles (arrow) and positive occipital sharp transients (POSTs).

Stage N2 sleep is defined by the presence of sleep spindles and K complexes. This stage has the same features as stage N1 with progressive slowing of background frequencies. Sleep spindles are transient, sinusoidal 12- to 14-Hz activity with waxing and waning amplitude seen in the central regions with frontal representation by slower frequencies of 10 to 12 Hz. A *K-complex* is a high amplitude diphasic wave with an initial sharp transient followed by a high-amplitude slow wave often associated with a sleep spindle in the frontocentral regions. A K-complex may be evoked by a sudden auditory stimulus. A persistent asymmetry of greater than 50% is abnormal on the side of reduction.

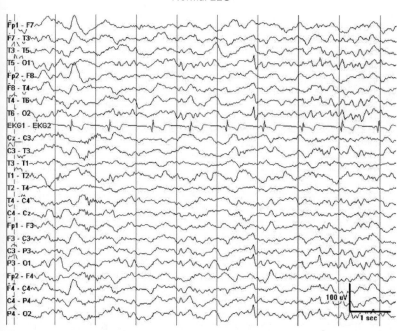

FIGURE 1.30. N3 sleep with prominent delta slow waves. Note the intermittent positive occipital sharp transients (POSTs) and sleep spindles against the continuous delta background.

Stage N3 (fka slow-wave sleep, slow sleep, delta sleep) best describes non-REM or deep sleep. It is comprised of 1- to 2-Hz delta frequencies occupying variable amounts of the background. Stage N3 contains delta waves occupying greater than 20% of the recording with voltages that are greater than 75 μV.

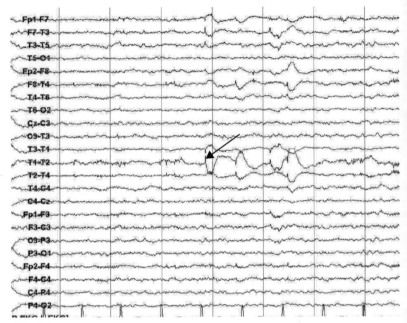

FIGURE 1.31. Prominent lateral rectus spikes (arrow) during rapid eye movement (REM) sleep. Spikes occur with rapid eye movements to the left, right, left, and right in the 4th to 6th second.

REM sleep is characterized by rapid eye movements, loss of muscle tone, and centrally-predominant saw-toothed waves in the EEG (Figure 1.31). Non-REM and REM sleep alternate in cycles four to six times during a normal night's sleep. A predominance of non-REM appears in the first part of the night, and REM in the last third of the night. A routine EEG with REM may reflect sleep deprivation and not necessarily reflect a disorder of sleep-onset REM such as narcolepsy.

ACTIVATION PROCEDURES

Activation techniques are a useful part of EEG in clinical practice and represent various types of stimuli or modalities that are able to trigger abnormalities. Hyperventilation and intermittent photic stimulation are routinely performed to augment slowing and/or epileptiform abnormalities, although sleep deprivation, pharmacological, and other methods may be employed.

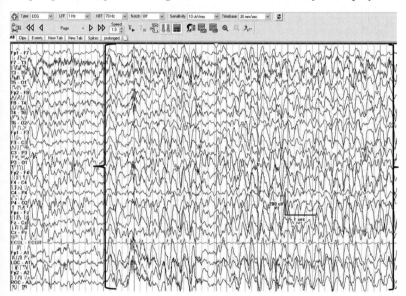

FIGURE 1.32. Normal build-up during hyperventilation. Note the frequently intermixed high amplitude delta (brackets) that occurs during wakefulness. The patient was a 16-year-old male who last ate greater than 12 hours before this EEG.

Hyperventilation is routinely performed for 2 to 3 minutes in most EEG laboratories. The purpose is to create cerebral vasoconstriction through a respiratory means of promoting systemic hypocarbia. Hyperventilation normally produces an intermittent to continuous bilateral increase in theta and delta frequencies (build-up) that is frontally dominant, and often high amplitude. Resolution of the effect occurs normally within 1 to 2 minutes.

(Continued)

Activation, or the generation of epileptiform discharges, is infrequently seen in those with localization-related epilepsy (less than 10%); however, this may approach 80% for those with genetic generalized epilepsies that include absence seizures. Hyperventilation may produce focal slowing in patients with an underlying structural lesion. It should not be performed in patients with severe cardiac or pulmonary disease, acute or recent stroke, significant large vessel cerebrovascular, and sickle cell anemia or trait, and it should be used with caution during pregnancy.

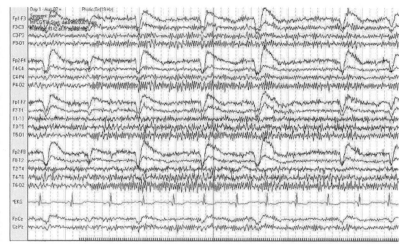

FIGURE 1.33. Photic driving at 20 Hz is best seen in the P3-O1, P4-O2, T5-O1, and T6-O2 derivations.

Intermittent photic stimulation normally produces potentials exquisitely time locked to the frequency of the intermittent light stimulus, and is referred to as *photic driving*. Response depends upon background illumination and the distance of the light source from the patient. Distances of less than 30 cm from the patient are used to optimize the effect of stimulation. Flashes are very brief, and delivered in sequence from 1 to 30 Hz flash frequencies for approximately 10 sec before stopping the stimulus. Subharmonics and harmonics of the flash frequency may be seen. Photic driving is usually greatest in the occipital location, in frequencies approximating the alpha rhythm, when the eyes are closed. *Photomyoclonic* (or *photomyogenic) responses* consist of a frontally dominant muscle artifact that occurs when the flash evokes repetitive local contraction of the frontalis musculature (photomyogenic). The periocular muscles may also be affected with single lightening-like head jerks (photomyoclonic). Myogenic spikes occurring 50 to 60 msec after the flash often increase in amplitude as the stimulus frequency increases and is more prolonged. This response is normal, although it may be seen as withdrawal syndromes or states of hyperexcitability.

BENIGN VARIANTS OF UNCERTAIN SIGNIFICANCE

Patterns that are rhythmic or epileptiform are often features that are associated with an abnormal EEG. Known patterns of uncertain significance or "benign variants" may possess these same characteristics and may reflect pitfalls for those interpreting EEG.

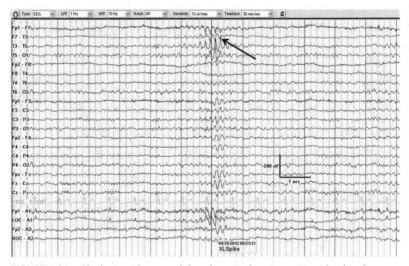

FIGURE 1.34. Rhythmic mid-temporal theta burst in drowsiness. Note the sharply contoured morphology of this burst of 6 Hz theta that is typical of this benign variant (arrow).

Rhythmic temporal theta bursts of drowsiness is now the preferred term for what was previously described as a psychomotor variant. This pattern occurs in 0.5% to 2.0% of selected normal adults and consists of bursts or runs of 5- to 7-Hz theta waves that may appear sharp, flat, or notched in appearance. It is maximal in the mid-temporal derivations and was referred to as rhythmic mid-temporal theta bursts of drowsiness. It is an interictal pattern that does not evolve spatially or temporally, although it may be represented bilaterally or independently over both hemispheres. It is seen in adolescents and adults in relaxed wakefulness.

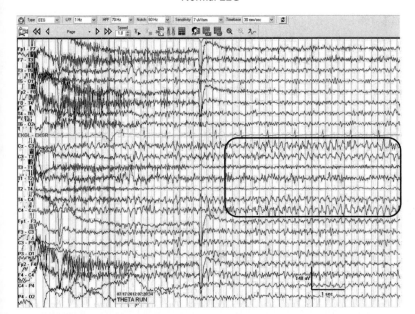

FIGURE 1.35. Central theta seen during the awake state in a 25-year-old female with multiple unexplained symptoms. Note the rhythmic sinusoidal 6 Hz theta (maximal at Cz; box) in this normal EEG.

A focal sinusoidal or arciform 4- to 7-Hz theta rhythm maximally expressed over the midline vertex region was first described by Ciganek. While morphologically it may resemble a mu rhythm, it is not similarly reactive, is slower in frequency, and occurs both in drowsiness and the wakefulness appearing morphologically as a rhythmic arciform, smooth, or sinusoidal rhythm. While initially Ciganek rhythm was felt to be a projected rhythm in temporal lobe epilepsy, it has since been seen in a heterogeneous population and is, therefore, considered a normal variant of uncertain clinical significance that is unrelated to epilepsy.

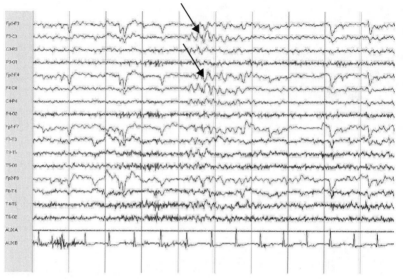

FIGURE 1.36. A 6-Hz (phantom) spike-wave burst (arrows) is seen with frontal predominance in the 5th second of this EEG in a patient with temporal lobe epilepsy. Note the low amplitude of the 6 Hz spike reflects the "phantom" portion of its name.

Spike-and-wave discharges at 6 Hz were first known as "phantom spike-and-waves." The acronyms WHAM (wakefulness, high amplitude, anterior, male) and FOLD (female, occipital, low amplitude, drowsy) were used to describe the two primary subtypes. Bilateral, synchronous, 6-Hz spike-and-wave discharges may range from 5 to 7 Hz, although with a typical repetition rate of 6 Hz lasting briefly for 1 to 2 sec. The spike is often of very low amplitude, at times difficult to appreciate during routine interpretation of the EEG by qualitative visual analysis. When the spikes are low amplitude and occur only during drowsiness, they usually represent a benign finding. When they are seen with high-amplitude spikes and occur with less than a 6-Hz frequency, or occur during wakefulness and persist into slow-wave sleep, there is a greater association with seizures.

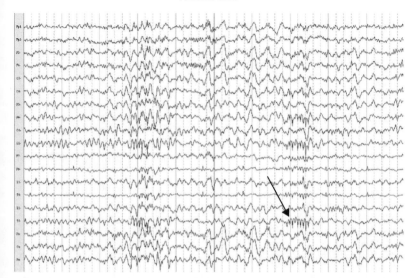

FIGURE 1.37. Fourteen- and 6-Hz positive bursts maximal in the T6 electrode derivation in a linked-ears reference montage. Note the downward deflection and prominent 14-Hz frequency (arrow).

Fourteen- and 6-Hz positive bursts (originally called 14- and 6-Hz positive spikes) have also been called ctenoids. They appear in the EEG in bursts of positive comb-like spindles mainly over the posterior temporal head regions. They are present most frequently at a rate of 14 or 6 to 7 Hz and last 0.5 to 1.0 sec in duration. The 14-Hz frequency is most prevalent, and the 6- Hz burst may appear with or without the faster frequencies. They are most common during adolescence, although they may persist into adulthood and decrease with age. The bursts are usually unilateral or bilaterally asynchronous with a shifting predominance involving one hemisphere to a greater degree. A contralateral ear reference montage and greater interelectrode distance best demonstrate these bursts.

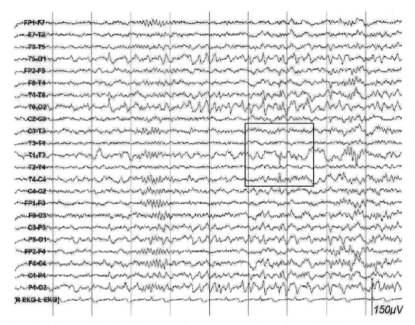

FIGURE 1.38. A right benign epileptiform transient of sleep (BETS) in the temporal region (box) during stage N2 sleep. Note the higher amplitude in the T1 and T2 channel with a longer interelectrode distance.

Different terms have been used to describe benign epileptiform transients of sleep (BETS). Previously known as mall sharp spikes and benign sporadic sleep spikes of sleep, BETS are typically depicted by a low-voltage (less than 50 µV), brief-duration (less than 50 msec), simple waveform with a monophasic or diphasic spike with a broad field that is absent in N3 sleep. Unlike the prior terms used to reflect BETS, their features on EEG may be greater than 50 µV, have a duration greater than 50 msec, and may appear with an aftergoing slow-wave (though usually of lower amplitude than the spike). This benign variant of uncertain significance has the morphology of a spike, although it has a rapidly ascending limb and steep descending limb, best seen in the anterior to mid-temporal derivations during N1 and N2 non-REM sleep. They are most common in adults. They are not associated with ipsilateral focal slowing and do not occur in runs. The most distinguishing characteristic is that they disappear in N3 sleep. They usually appear as a unilateral discharge, but are almost always independent when they are bilateral. They possess a field that may correspond to an oblique transverse dipole, resulting in opposite polarities seen in different hemispheres when they are bilateral.

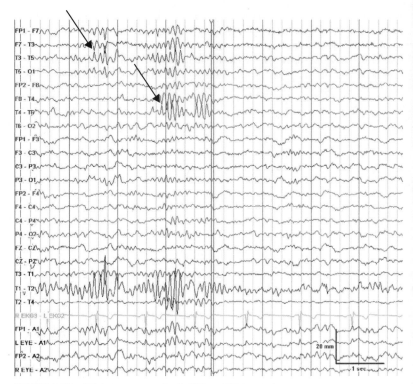

FIGURE 1.39. Wicket waves maximal at T3 and T4 (arrows).

Wicket spikes are most commonly seen in adults over 30. They occur within the 6- to 11-Hz band, and can obtain amplitudes of up to 200 µV. They are seen over the temporal regions during drowsiness and light sleep and are usually bilateral and independent. They typically occur in bursts, although they may be confused with IEDs, especially when they occur independently or as isolated waveforms. No focal slowing or aftergoing slow-wave component is seen, and they likely represent fragmented temporal alpha activity. Similar frequency and morphology of the bursts, if compared to the isolated waveforms, is a means of providing support for their nonepileptogenic origin. Wicket waves are considered an epileptiform normal variant though they are commonly mistaken as abnormal sharp waves resulting in misdiagnosis.

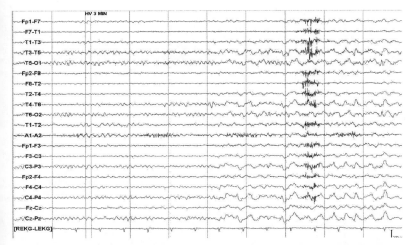

FIGURE 1.40. Subclinical rhythmic electrographic discharge in adults (SREDA) present in a 73-year-old patient that occurred during hyperventilation (HV). No clinical signs were present.

In contrast to many of the patterns of uncertain significance that mimic IEDs, subclinical rhythmic electrographic discharge in adults (SREDA) is a pattern that mimics the epileptiform characteristics of a subclinical seizure. However, no clinical features exist during it, either subjective or objective findings, and no association with epilepsy has been demonstrated. In contrast to most benign variants, SREDA is more likely to occur in those over 50 and also while the person is awake. It may exist in two forms, either as a bilateral episodic burst of rhythmic, sharply contoured 5- to 7-Hz theta frequencies appearing maximal over the temporoparietal derivations or as an abrupt mononphasic series of repetitive sharp or slow waveforms that appear focally at the vertex, recurring in progressively shorter intervals until a sustained burst is noted. Rarely, the two forms may appear in the same person. Bursts of SREDA usually last between 40 and 80 sec and occur without postictal slowing.

(Continued)

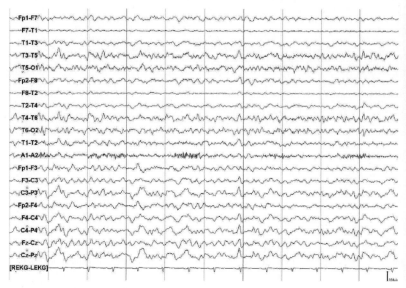

FIGURE 1.40. (Continued)

ADDITIONAL RESOURCES

Abou-Khalil B, Misulis KE. *Atlas of EEG and Seizure Semiology*. Philadelphia, PA: Butterworth Heinemann; 2006:1-213.

Benbadis SR, Tatum WO. Overinterpretation of EEGs and misdiagnosis of epilepsy. *J Clin Neurophysiol*. 2003;20:42-44.

Blume WT, Masako K, Young GB. *Atlas of Adult Electroencephalography*. 2nd ed. Philadelphia, PA: Lippincott Williams & Wilkins; 2002:1-531.

Kellaway P. Orderly approach to visual analysis: elements of the normal EEG and their characteristics in children and adults. In: Ebersole JS, Pedley TA, eds. *Current Practice of Clinical Electroencephalography*. 3rd ed. Philadelphia, PA: Lippincott Williams & Wilkins; 2003:100-159.

Markand ON. Pearls, perils, and pitfalls in the use of the electroencephalogram. *Semin Neurol*. 2003;23(1):7-46.

Olejniczak P. Neurophysiologic basis of EEG. *J Clin Neurophysiol*. 2006;23(3):186-189.

Tatum WO IV, Husain AM, Benbadis SR, Kaplan PW. Normal human adult EEG and normal variants. *J Clin Neurophysiol*. 2006;23(3):194-207.

Tatum WO. Artifact-related epilepsy. *Neurology*. 2013;80 (suppl 1):S12-S25.

Tatum WO. EEG interpretation: common problems. *Clin Pract*. 2012;9(5):527-538.

Tatum WO. Normal "Suspicious" EEG. *Neurology*. 2013;80(1)(suppl 1):S4-S11.

Westmoreland BF. Benign electroencephalographic variants and patterns of uncertain clinical significance. In: Ebersole JS, Pedley TA, eds. *Current Practice of Clinical Electroencephalography*. 3rd ed. Philadelphia, PA: Lippincott Williams & Wilkins; 2003:235-245.

2

Abnormal Nonepileptiform EEG

Selim R. Benbadis

Interictal EEG provides useful information about the presence of non-epileptiform neurophysiological dysfunction. When abnormalities are encountered, they are not specific for an underlying etiology, and as such represent abnormalities without further differentiation of the pathological process. While neuroimaging demonstrates anatomical definition of an abnormality, the EEG provides evidence of abnormal neurophysiological function when neuroimaging is normal.

The EEG is sensitive to cerebral dysfunction, but may have a lag during clinical improvement or lead relative to maximal clinical symptomatology. Many of the patterns that are nonepileptiform are due to a nonspecific etiology. Still, the presence of a nonepileptiform abnormality reflects the clinical presence of abnormality and often parallels the degree of dysfunction. Acuity is unable to be demonstrated by EEG in nonepileptiform abnormalities, although serial tracing may further help to define the trend of neurological improvement or deterioration. Therefore, the EEG is objectively able to substantiate and quantify the degree or depth of encephalopathy when diffuse nonepileptiform abnormalities are encountered. Furthermore, they may lateralize (or even localize) abnormalities when focal areas of slowing are evident. Many nonepileptiform and epileptiform abnormalities may help characterize the encephalopathy when the two features are identified on the EEG. This chapter will discuss and focus on generalized and focal nonepileptiform abnormalities.

DIFFUSE SLOWING

Diffuse slowing on the EEG may have various morphologies, and occur intermittently or continuously, to reflect abnormal cerebral function. The presence of diffuse slowing suggests a bilateral disturbance of cerebral function and represents an encephalopathy that is nonspecific for etiology.

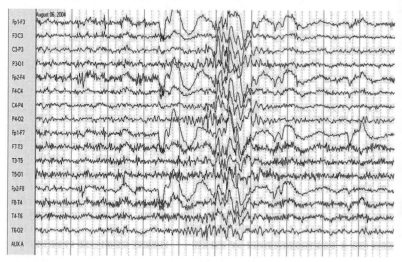

FIGURE 2.1. An abnormal high-amplitude burst of diffuse intermittent theta in an awake adult following a motor vehicle accident associated with driving under the influence.

Intermixed diffuse intermittent theta in the most alert state is normal in young adults. When theta frequencies are seen in the frontal or frontocentral regions and voltages are greater than 100 µV or when theta is present greater than 10% of the time in an adult (not in childhood or elderly), then theta may reflect a nonspecific abnormality similar to diffuse intermittent slowing or background slowing, but may be seen normally in young adults. The slower the frequency, the higher the amplitude, and the greater the persistence, the more likely intermittent theta is abnormal.

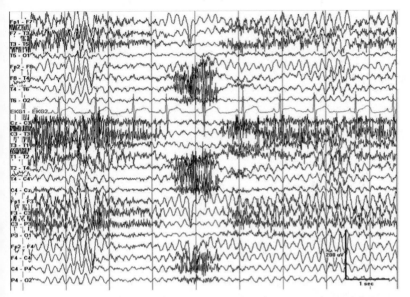

FIGURE 2.2. Generalized monomorphic 5- to 6-Hz theta frequencies obtained during a syncopal episode in a patient undergoing head-up tilt table testing for neurocardiogenic syncope.

Diffuse (or generalized) slowing of the background electrocerebral activity reflects a nonspecific abnormality. It is indicative of a bilateral disturbance of cerebral function. With progression of cerebral dysfunction, the degree of generalized abnormal nonepileptiform abnormalities increases. Abnormally intermixed intermittent slowing that is manifest initially as intermittent theta (sometimes normal as discussed above) progresses to involve a greater degree of intermittent slowing first becoming continuous theta slowing that is subsequently replaced by greater amounts of higher amplitude delta frequencies.

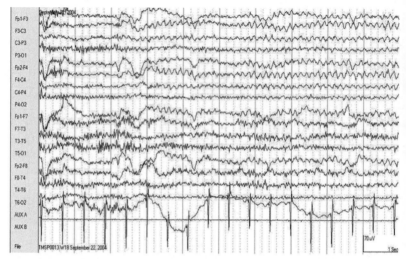

FIGURE 2.3. EEG demonstrating diffuse slowing of the posterior dominant rhythm to 6 Hz. This degree of slowing of a well-defined background is abnormally slow even in a 65-year-old man.

Background slowing is defined as slowing of the posterior background activity to a frequency slower than the normal alpha rhythm frequency of 8 Hz. Diffuse slowing of the posterior dominant rhythm is a feature of encephalopathy. The degree of slowing of the background reflects the degree of cerebral dysfunction. A greater degree of background slowing reflects a more severe encephalopathy. Abnormality is defined when a posterior dominant rhythm that is present that is normally reactive appears too slow for the patient's age. The lower limits of normal for an alpha rhythm is 5, 6, 7, and 8 Hz at ages 1, 3, 5, and 8 years old, respectively. Often times, diffuse slowing of the background is associated with other stigmata of mild diffuse encephalopathy such as intermittent bursts of generalized theta or delta activity.

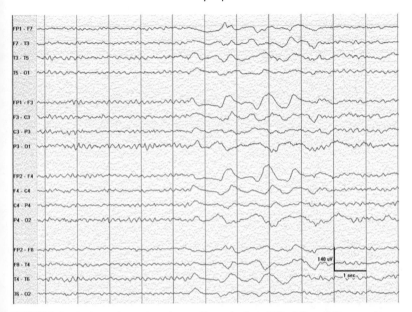

FIGURE 2.4. An intermittent 4-sec burst of irregular 1- to 2-Hz delta activity occurring on a diffusely slow posterior dominant rhythm of 6 Hz. This 55-year-old woman was clinically confused and disoriented, with multiple metabolic and systemic disturbances.

Diffuse intermittent slowing is characterized by intermittent bursts of diffuse slow activity. This usually appears in the delta range and often appears in addition to background slowing of the posterior dominant rhythm (see above). Like background slowing, with which it frequently coexists, it is indicative of a diffuse encephalopathy. The bursts are usually irregular or polymorphic but can occasionally be rhythmic. As the severity of the encephalopathy increases, the bursts will increase in duration and frequency and merge into or become continuous generalized slowing (see continuous generalized slowing, page 60). Like other encephalopathic patterns, the presence of diffuse intermittent slowing is nonspecific relative to an etiology and may reflect either the presence of cortical or subcortical cerebral dysfunction.

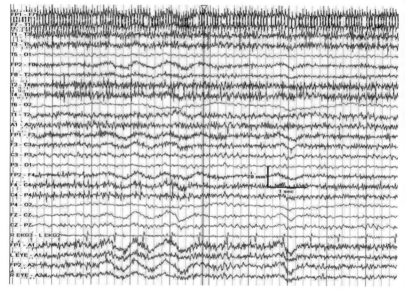

FIGURE 2.5. Frontal intermittent rhythmic delta activity in a 67-year-old patient with noncommunicating hydrocephalus. Note the slower 1.0- to 1.5-Hz frequency and the cerebral origin that is verified by the eye movement monitors.

Frontal intermittent rhythmic delta activity (FIRDA) appears as bursts of intermittent delta. These intermittent bursts are often high voltage, bisynchronous, and monomorphic waveforms. FIRDA may rarely appear asymmetric, especially when a focal structural lesion is present. However, FIRDA typically has a bilaterally symmetric electrophysiological field. FIRDA may appear normally during the build-up associated with hyperventilation (see Chapter 1). An abnormal pattern exists when FIRDA occurs in the waking adult EEG consisting of bilateral rhythmic monomorphic delta waves. The frequency is usually consistent throughout the EEG when it appears. Bifrontal predominance is typical in adults, and occipital predominance is more typically seen in children shifting with brain maturation. FIRDA is most often associated with encephalopathies of toxic or metabolic origin. It also occurs with subcortical lesions such as a deep midline lesion or increased intracranial pressure (above).

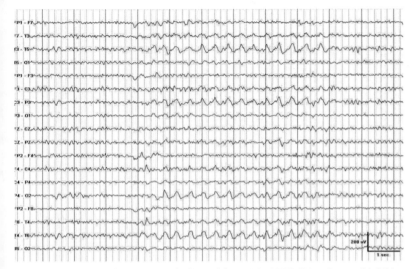

FIGURE 2.6. Occipital intermittent rhythmic delta activity (ORIDA) in a 6-year-old child with absence epilepsy.

Occipital intermittent rhythmic delta activity (OIRDA), like FIRDA, is a nonspecific finding in the EEG relative to etiology. OIRDA is demonstrated as a posterior predominant bisynchronous rhythmic delta slowing appearing in bursts. OIRDA has the same features as FIRDA, but occurs in children. OIRDA appears maximal over the occipital region instead of appearing with frontal predominance. OIRDA has been noted to occur in association with generalized (absence) epilepsy, but is not an epileptiform abnormality unless intermixed spikes are present.

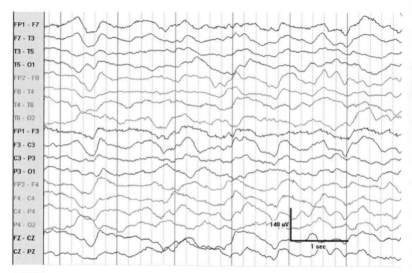

FIGURE 2.7. Continuous irregular 1.5- to 3.0-Hz delta in a 66-year-old man with encephalopathy that was unresponsive. The above sample of EEG was representative of the entire record. No reactivity of the background was present during the EEG.

Continuous generalized slowing consists of polymorphic delta activity that is continuous or near-continuous (greater than 80% of the record) and (at least as importantly) unreactive. *Unreactive* implies no change in the background electrocerebral activity produced with external stimuli in addition to the absence of sleep-wake patterns. Unlike the prior two examples of background slowing and intermittent generalized slowing, continuous generalized unreactive polymorphic delta slowing is indicative of a severe diffuse encephalopathy. Most patients with this feature are comatose or stuporous. Like the other nonepileptiform abnormalities associated with encephalopathy, this finding is nonspecific as to etiology. The most common causes by far are toxic-metabolic or systemic disturbances. However, severe diffuse, bilateral structural lesions or injury affecting the brain can also produce this pattern (e.g., traumatic brain injuries or advanced neurodegenerative diseases).

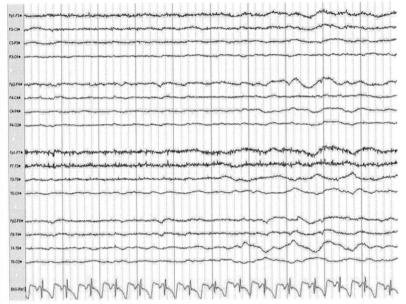

FIGURE 2.8. Low-voltage recording in a patient involved in a motor vehicle accident. The recording was obtained at a sensitivity of 2 μV/mm with no waveforms demonstrating a voltage of greater than 20 μV.

Low-voltage EEG is typically associated with diffuse slowing of the background rhythm. In general, the state of the patient is the best indicator of abnormality with some low-voltage EEGs of less than 10 to 20 μV found in a subset of normal individuals. When seen during encephalopathy or coma, low-voltage EEG is typically associated with diffuse slowing and poor reactivity to somatosensory stimulation. One distinguishing characteristic is the lack of admixed alpha and beta frequencies in this low-voltage recording.

FOCAL ABNORMALITIES

Focal abnormalities on the EEG provide electrographic evidence of a localized abnormal cerebral function. They are not specific for etiology and may be seen with many different underlying structural lesions that affect the brain. They may also be encountered as a temporary nonstructural physiological effect (i.e., following a seizure). The location, morphology, persistence, and poor reactivity are features that suggest an underlying structural lesion, but because the specificity is low, a broad differential is required.

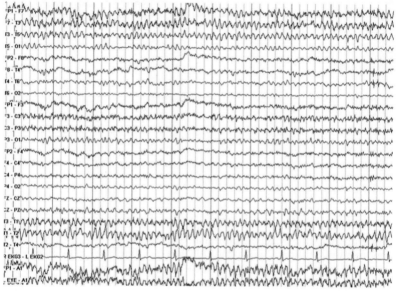

FIGURE 2.9A. Alpha asymmetry in a patient with an acute right fronto-parietal ischemic infarction.

(Continued)

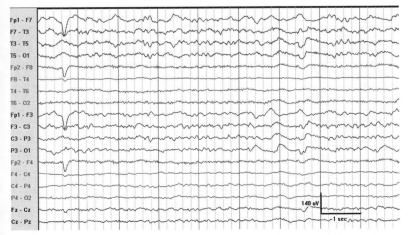

FIGURE 2.9B. Right hemisphere suppression in a patient with a right hemisphere intracerebral hemorrhage. Note the dramatic difference in amplitude.

Alpha asymmetries depict an abnormality on the side ipsilateral to the hemisphere and characteristically involve a slow posterior dominant rhythm. Additional focal, regional, or lateralized abnormalities are often seen in conjunction with alpha asymmetries. A persistent hemispheric difference of greater than 1 Hz should be regarded as being abnormal when alpha asymmetry is seen. Additionally, while the right hemisphere is often normally asymmetrical with respect to the amplitude, a persistent amplitude asymmetry of greater than 50% should be regarded as abnormal.

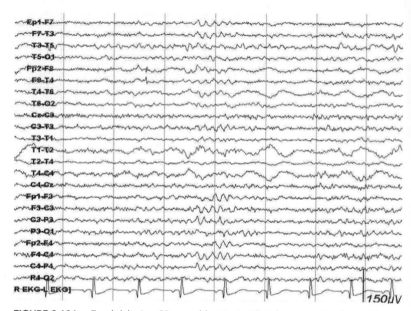

FIGURE 2.10A. Focal delta in a 28-year-old patient with right temporal polymorphic delta due to an anterior temporal ganglioglioma. Note the anterior-mid-temporal localization with loss of the intermixed faster frequencies.

Focal polymorphic delta is confined to one or two electrode contacts and indicates a more restricted disturbance of cerebral dysfunction affecting the white matter tracts. When concomitant loss of faster frequencies is seen (above), these findings on the EEG may be more suggestive of a structural lesion that affects both the ipsilateral gray and white matter of the hemisphere. The more focal and persistent the polymorphic delta slowing, the greater the likelihood a structural lesion will be present. Continuous regional delta slowing may also appear on invasive EEG with the same frequencies represented as scalp recording.

(Continued)

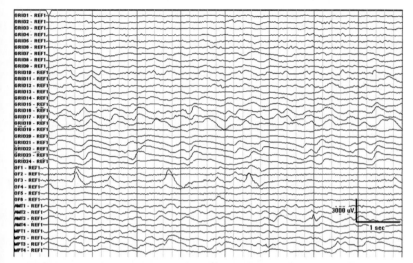

FIGURE 2.10B. Sample of intracranial EEG using subdural electrodes. Note the focal slow (delta) activity at contacts OF3, grid 22-24, and grid 16-18. Rules for localization are similar on invasive recordings, and on referential montages this indicates a focal area of dysfunction found to be caused by a small hemorrhage.

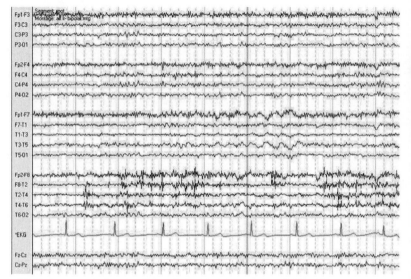

FIGURE 2.11. Temporal intermittent rhythmic delta activity (TIRDA) in a patient with left temporal lobe epilepsy. Note the brief burst of regional bisynchronous bitemporal TIRDA (line).

Temporal intermittent rhythmic delta activity (TIRDA) is a unique form of intermittent rhythmic delta activity. It consists of intermittent monomorphic focal bursts of monomorphic delta frequencies maximal typically in a unilateral temporal derivation. The presence of TIRDA has a strong association with focal seizures. It may provide localizing capabilities in patients with temporal lobe epilepsy. TIRDA is often associated with interictal epileptiform discharges (IEDs) and is abnormal when it occurs during the awake state and is persistent.

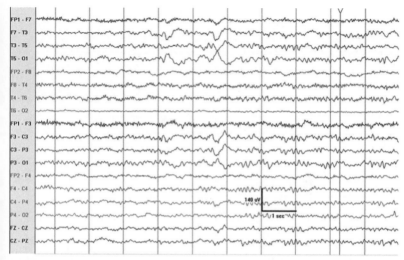

FIGURE 2.12. There is a brief 2-sec burst of polymorphic delta activity in the posterior temporal-parietal region of the left hemisphere in a 55-year-old patient with a left subcortical white matter lacunar infarction.

Intermittent irregular slowing has a low correlation with an underlying lesion compared to focal slowing that is continuous. Focal slowing may indicate an underlying structural lesion involving the white matter tracts of the brain. Definite statements about the specific etiology due to the intermittent irregular slow activity cannot be derived by the appearance of the EEG as with most nonepileptiform abnormalities.

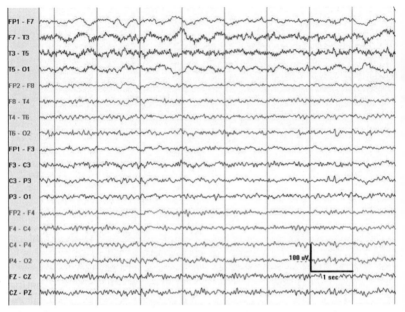

FIGURE 2.13A. A 75-year-old patient with an acute left frontal ischemic infarct. Note the left hemispheric temporally-predominant polymorphic delta that affects the entire hemisphere.

Continuous regional delta slowing on the EEG has a high correlation with an underlying structural lesion involving the white matter of the ipsilateral hemisphere. The area of slowing usually overlies the hemisphere containing the structural lesion, but does not necessarily reflect the precise location as the one represented by EEG. For example, frontal lobe lesions may appear as ipsilateral continuous regional delta slowing on EEG. Trauma, tumor, stroke, intracranial hemorrhages, and infection all create a similar appearance on the EEG without specific features. The EEG may be abnormal and demonstrate continuous regional delta slowing that indicates a reversible structural lesion with resolution.

(Continued)

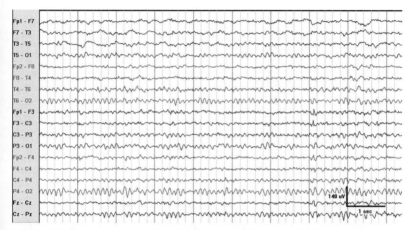

FIGURE 2.13B. Typical focal or "regional" (not hemispheric) slowing in a patient with transient aphasia but no stroke on imaging. The delta activity is present in the left frontotemporal region, but not in the paracentral area. In the absence of a structural abnormality (MRI), the patient was felt to have had a transient ischemic attack (TIA), or less likely a seizure with postictal state.

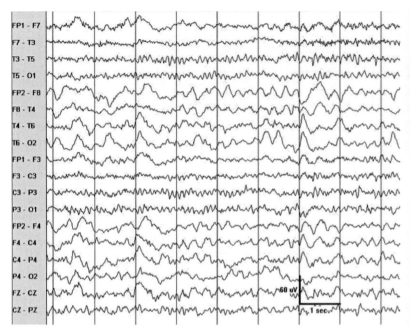

FIGURE 2.14A. This EEG was taken from a 64-year-old after a right hemisphere ischemic infarct. Note that a well-formed alpha rhythm is not present in the right hemisphere compared with the left and is instead replaced by continuous right hemispheric polymorphic delta slowing.

Lateralized polymorphic delta slowing may consist of theta or delta frequencies that are focal, regional, or lateralized. Delta that is polymorphic (and arrhythmic) is composed of slow-wave activity that is 3.5 Hz (or less) and is composed of waveforms that vary in frequency and duration. Polymorphic delta activity when localized is indicative of an underlying supratentorial lesion affecting the white matter of the ipsilateral hemisphere. The more state-independent and persistent the delta slowing appears, the greater the likelihood that a structural lesion will be present. Lateralized

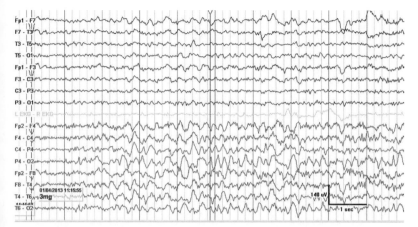

FIGURE 2.14B. Right hemisphere slow activity induced by intracarotid methohexital (3 mg) during a Wada test. This illustrates typical "focal" (lateralized) dysfunction. This only lasts a few minutes due to the short half-life of methohexital.

or even localized polymorphic delta, however, may be seen as a transitory phenomenon on the EEG due to head injury, transient ischemic attack, migraine, and during a postictal state. Iatrogenic causes such as the intracarotid amobarbital procedure (Wada test) may also produce hemispheric slowing due to the transitory effects attempting to produce hemi-anesthesia used for presurgical lateralization of language and memory function.

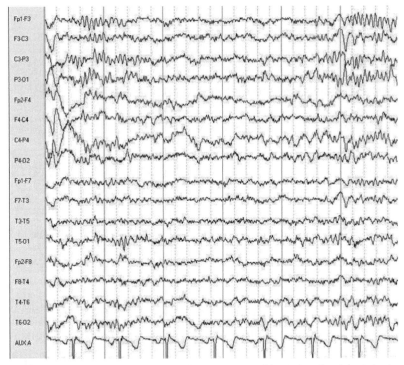

FIGURE 2.15. Asymmetry of sleep spindles in a 36-year-old patient with a right thalamic glioma.

Sleep spindles are initially evident in the first 2 months, and by 2 years of age are synchronous in normal children. Sleep elements are normally maximal in frequency in the central location, although they may appear in the frontal regions as well. A frequency of 12 to 14 Hz is observed in the central regions and is the distinguishing characteristic of stage N2 sleep. Spindles are very stable in their bilateral appearance and a persistent slowing of the spindle frequency or the unilateral appearance of sleep spindles should be regarded as an abnormal nonepileptiform feature.

ADDITIONAL RESOURCES

Benbadis SR. Focal disturbances of brain function. In: Levin KH, Lüders HO, eds. *Comprehensive Clinical Neurophysiology*. Philadelphia, PA: Saunders; 2000;457-467.

Epstein CM, Riecher AM, Henderson RM, et al. EEG in liver transplantation: visual and computerized analysis. *Electroencephalogr Clin Neurophysiol*. 1992;83:367-371.

Gloor P, Kalabay O, Giard N. The electroencephalogram in diffuse encephalopathies: electroenephalographic correlates of gray and white matter lesions. *Brain* 1968;91:779-802.

Kaplan PW. Metabolic and endocrine disorders resembling seizures. In: Engel J Jr, Pedley TA, eds. *Epilepsy: A Comprehensive Textbook*. Philadelphia, PA: Lippincott Raven; 1997:2661-2670.

Liporace J, Tatum W, Morris GL, et al. Clinical utility of sleep-deprived versus computer-assisted ambulatory 16-channel EEG in epilepsy patients: a multicenter study. *Epilepsy Res*. 1998;32:357-362.

Luders H, Noachtar S, eds. *Atlas and Classification of Electroencephalography*. Philadelphia, PA: Saunders; 2000.

Schaul N, Gloor P, Gotman J. The EEG in deep midline lesions. *Neurology* 1981;31:157-167.

Zifkin BG, Cracco RQ. An orderly approach to the abnormal electroencephalogram. In: Ebersole JS, Pedley TA, eds. *Current Practice of Clinical Electroencephalography*. 3rd ed. Philadelphia, PA: Lippincott Williams & Wilkins; 2003:288-302.

3

Interictal Epileptiform Discharges

William O. Tatum, IV

Interictal epileptiform discharges (IEDs) represent a distinct group of waveforms that are characteristically seen in persons with epilepsy. Variations of normal background rhythms, a variety of artifacts, and variants of uncertain significance may mimic abnormal IEDs and lead to over-interpretation of the electroencephalography (EEG) and untoward patient consequences (Chapter 1). IEDs have reliably been associated with epilepsy at rates sufficient enough to be clinically relevant and useful. Although prominent intrapatient and interpatient variability in frequency and morphology of IEDs may occur, those patients with prominent IEDs on the EEG are not necessarily the patients with more severe epilepsy. Scalp detection of IEDs is based upon dipole localization and the surrounding field. The resultant scalp detection of the source may appear different on the scalp EEG than the actual site of the seizure onset zone. In most cases, an IED reflects a radial dipole that is oriented to be detected on the scalp. However, tangential dipoles may commonly occur in certain epilepsy syndromes (e.g., benign childhood epilepsy with centrotemporal spikes [BCECTS]) and from developmentally or surgically altered cortex may produce unusual dipoles that challenge the EEG reader. Horizontal dipoles are better detected by magnetoencephalography which is a neurophysiologic test that is often complimentary to EEG in determining source localization. Rarely, normal individuals may possess IEDs on EEG without the phenotypic expression of seizures. The photoparoxysmal (PPR) response, generalized spike-and-waves (GSW), and centrotemporal IEDs are the most frequent asymptomatic IEDs. When they are encountered, they typically reflect the genotype of an inherited trait that is represented on the EEG without the phenotypic expression of clinical seizures. Additionally, focal IEDs have a variable association with clinical epilepsy and depend upon the location of their appearance. For example, central, parietal, and occipital spikes, in general, may be less likely to be associated with clinical epilepsy than IEDs associated with the frontal and temporal location in the absence of a structural lesion. IEDs have been seen in migraine, certain drugs such as lithium or clozapine, the austistic spectrum disorder, cerebral palsy, and blindness among others.

The interictal EEG plays a pivotal role in providing ancillary support for a clinical diagnosis of epilepsy. The presence of abnormal IEDs occurs in less than 1% to 2% of normal individuals. When IEDs are present in the interictal EEG, they can help to classify the type of seizure, the type of epilepsy, or the epilepsy syndrome. EEG support of the clinical diagnosis is provided by identifying the mechanism that would apply to the patients particular clinical semiology or semiologies (e.g., epilepsy with generalized tonic-clonic [GTC] seizures). Differentiating the epilepsies are based upon distinguishing seizures that have a focal onset in localization-related from those that are generalized in onset facilitated by the type and distribution of IEDs noted on the EEG. Focal IEDs may be either focal, regional, lateralized, or secondarily generalized discharges (aka secondary bilateral synchrony [SBS] on EEG) and are characterized by their field of involvement. Their presence may help provide information that is useful in localizing the epileptogenic zone for the purposes of surgical treatment. Frontal, anterior temporal, and midline IEDs have the highest correlation with seizures. Furthermore, there is treatment information that can be clinically relevant in following the response to therapy (e.g., as in the case of the medical management of absence seizures). In addition IEDs may provide prognostic information when considering a trial of antiepileptic drug taper and signify a lower likelihood of success when persistent IEDs are evident on the EEG prior to tapering. In the absence of IEDs, epilepsy is not excluded because of the deep cortex, fissures, gyri, and sulcal neuroanatomy that may not readily be represented at the scalp during routine recording. The EEG, while ideally suited for evaluating patients with epilepsy, is also not specific for etiology when demonstrating IEDs. The scalp EEG may demonstrate similar interictal and ictal (Chapter 4) discharges, appearing in the same or different regions of the brain. While various morphologies of IEDs exist, their distribution usually implies one type of epilepsy as opposed to more than one type (e.g., focal and generalized epilepsy).

FOCAL EPILEPTIFORM DISCHARGES

Abnormal focal IEDs on EEG represent a heightened predisposition for the expression of focal seizures. The location of the focal IEDs varies with respect to the potential for the brain to generate clinical seizures and also implies what the behavioral manifestations are likely to be.

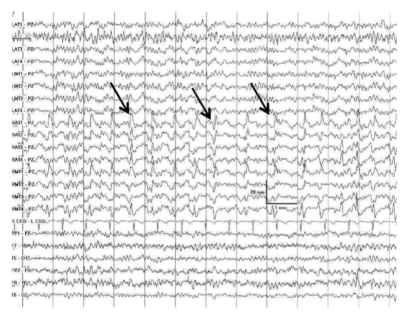

FIGURE 3.1. Intracranial (top 16 channels) and simultaneous scalp EEG recording (bottom 6 channels) obtained during a presurgical evaluation for drug-resistant epilepsy. Sensitivities in the top channels are 75 μv versus 7 μv/mm at the scalp. Note the absence of IEDs in the scalp EEG compared to the intracranial EEG where they occur at 1/sec (arrows).

It is often said that the presence of a normal interictal EEG does not exclude a clinical diagnosis of epilepsy. The cortex sampled by surface-based scalp EEG is an incomplete representation of the entire brain. Many deep-seated cortical gyri are unable to be "seen" unless intracranial electrodes are placed directly into or on top of the underlying cortex. Because scalp potentials are volume-conducted potentials through cerebrospinal fluid and meninges, skull, and subcutaneous tissue of the scalp, "buried" or low-amplitude potentials may be underrepresented at the level of the scalp EEG. Therefore, difficulty with source detection at the level of the scalp may arise because the generators of the IEDs are deep-seated (i.e., mesial frontal), small regions of involved cortex, exhibit rapid cortical propagation, or are obscured by movement or myogenic artifact.

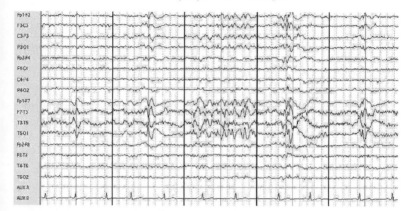

FIGURE 3.2. Different morphologies that occur with IEDs include sharp waves (seen during seconds 1 and 2), mixed spikes and sharp waves (in second 3), polyspike-and-slow waves (in second 4), and spike-and-wave discharges (in the last second of the figure). The above example was recorded during an ambulatory EEG in a patient with localization-related epilepsy.

Epileptiform discharges appear in different morphologies. Both *spikes* and *sharp waves* are referred to as IEDs (transients) and are defined by their duration. They are clearly distinguished from the background rhythm but have no difference with respect to epileptogenicity. A spike has a duration of 20 to 70 msec while a sharp wave lasts 70 to 200 msec and appears more "blunted" and can occur with or without an after-going slow wave. *Polyspikes* (or multispikes) are another common type of IED. Combinations of IEDs often occur in the same patient at different times (see Figure 3.2 above). Both spikes and sharp waves are generated at the top of the cortical gyrus and have a polarity that is most often negative at the surface of the human scalp EEG.

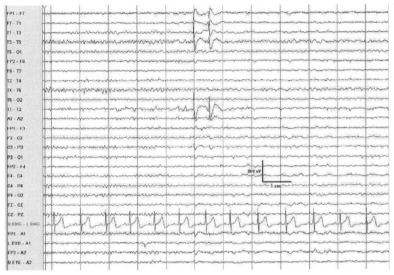

FIGURE 3.3. EEG demonstrating a couplet of left anterior temporal spike-and-slow waves. Note the very brief duration of approximately 20 msec.

Focal IEDs include epileptiform "spikes" that imply that a focal mechanism exists in a patient with a clinical diagnosis of epilepsy or seizures. The polarity of an abnormal epileptiform discharge designated as a spike is very frequently negative at the surface of the scalp EEG with a duration of 20 to 70 msec. Those discharges of less than 20 msec are suspicious for noncerebral potentials such as artifact that is generated by muscles. There may or may not be an after-going slow wave discharge. The location usually determines the potential for epileptogenicity with temporal locations usually carrying the highest association with clinical seizure expression. Furthermore, the seizure semiology can be inferred with anterior temporal IEDs carrying a greater risk for the expression of focal seizures of temporal lobe origin.

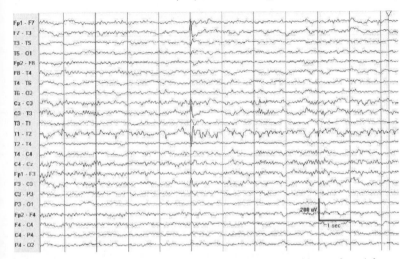

FIGURE 3.4. Left temporal sharp waves in the EEG of a 43-year-old man after a left temporal lobectomy who was being evaluated for reoperation. Note the positive phase reversal at T3.

Positive spikes are rarely encountered in the routine clinical EEG. IEDs (spikes and sharp waves) are almost always surface negative, generating the typical negative phase reversal in a bipolar montage. The situation encountered most commonly in clinical practice when positive polarity of the IEDs are seen occurs in patients who have had surgery and have an altered cortical anatomy (e.g., cortical dysplasia). In neonatal EEG, positive IEDs reflect periventricular injury and are not uncommon, although with development, unless congenital brain malformations are evident, positive sharp waves are rarely encountered in the adult EEG.

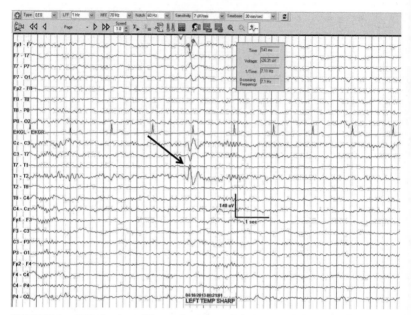

FIGURE 3.5. EEG showing a left anterior temporal sharp wave during second 5 (arrow) in a patient with drug-resistant temporal lobe epilepsy due to hippocampal sclerosis. Note the parameters of the sharp wave in the box.

The degree of epileptogenicity varies with location, but the temporal region is the most common epileptogenic region in the brain. Anterior temporal spikes or sharp waves often have a clinical association with focal seizures of temporal lobe origin more than 90% of the time. These discharges have maximal electronegativity at the F7/F8 derivations using the 10 to 20 system of electrode placement. However, the amplitude of these IEDs is usually greatest in the "true temporal" (at T1 and T2), ear, or sphenoidal electrodes when additional electrodes are utilized. In one-third of patients, the discharges are seen bilaterally, are activated by sleep, and localize best in wakefulness or rapid eye movement (REM) sleep when present.

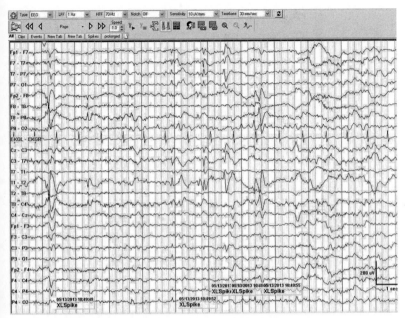

FIGURE 3.6. Bitemporal interictal epileptiform discharges maximal in the mid-temporal derivations in a patient with neocortical temporal lobe epilepsy.

Mid-temporal IEDs also occur in patients with temporal lobe epilepsy (TLE). In general, mid-temporal IEDs are often more regional in distribution and are more likely to be associated with lateral temporal neocortical epilepsy. Focal slowing and the presence of bilateral discharges appear more likely to be represented.

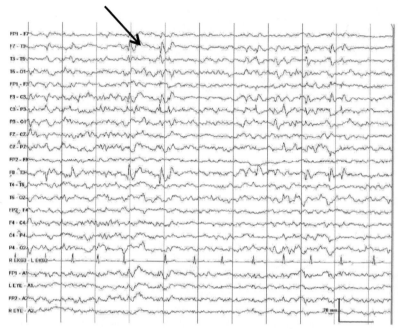

FIGURE 3.7. Left centrotemporal spikes (arrow) in a patient with BCECTS. Notice the central field of spread of the spikes and low-amplitude right frontal positivity.

Benign childhood epilepsy with centrotemporal spikes (BCECTS aka "Rolandic epilepsy") is a common childhood genetic localization-related epilepsy (LRE) syndrome. In this case, prominent centrotemporal IEDs are encountered with a characteristic diphasic morphology composed of a negative peak followed by a positive rounded component. This dipole characteristically reveals a maximum negativity in the centrotemporal region. When a contralateral maximum positivity in the frontal (or vertex) region is seen, this characterizes the tangential dipole of BCECTS. Spikes are markedly activated during non-REM sleep with the dipole best demonstrated on referential montages.

This contralateral positivity has been used to separate the more "benign" nature of BCECTs from a more pathological rolandic sharp wave (e.g., Landau–Kleffner syndrome of acquired epileptic aphasia and those with LRE).

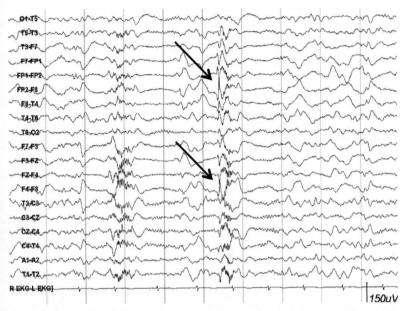

FIGURE 3.8. A right frontal spike and polyspike signified by the phase reversals (arrows) during a secondary bilateral synchronous discharge in a patient with frontal lobe epilepsy.

Frontal spikes are often found in patients with frontal lobe epilepsy (FLE), although they may be absent in up to one-third of patients. They may also appear as fragmented GSW discharges in Genetic Generalized epilepsy (GGE) during drowsiness. The IEDs of FLE are often spikes with high-amplitude broad discharges that may be reflected in the contralateral frontal region. IEDs or slowing may be best seen independently over the frontal and frontal-polar regions when orbital frontal seizures occur. SBS or diffuse discharges arising from a focal point in the frontal lobe (Figures 3.8 and 3.14) may occur in up to two-thirds of individuals with FLE. Transverse montages are best to distinguish a lateralized generator from two discrete bisynchronous generators.

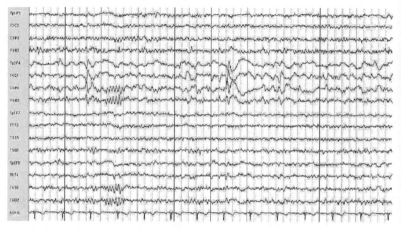

FIGURE 3.9. Right central spike-and-slow wave IEDs and focal slowing in a patient with a right posterior frontal brain tumor and recurrent focal seizures.

Central IEDs can occur with the symptomatic LREs at any age. Overall, central IEDs are less frequently associated with epilepsy than those arising from temporal or frontal lobe origin. Some conditions may give rise to central spikes without epilepsy and include cerebral palsy, migraine, and those seen as an inherited trait without seizures (e.g., siblings of those with BCECTS). In addition, some normal features of the EEG (e.g., fragmented mu rhythm) can mimic abnormal central IEDs. However, unlike normal rhythms (e.g., mu rhythms), abnormal central IEDs often have a quicker "rise" on the upstroke of the discharge, may be associated with an after-going slow wave, occur in a state independent fashion (not just drowsiness and light sleep), and/or be associated with focal slowing in the same region.

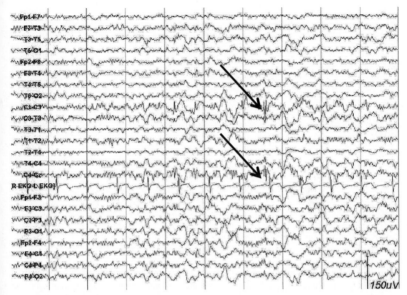

FIGURE 3.10. Midline Cz spikes (arrows) in a patient with frontal lobe epilepsy. These Cz spikes were identified in the waking and deep sleep states to distinguish them as pathological.

Midline spikes may occur at Cz, Fz, and Pz and are seen more frequently in children, but may also occur in adults. Isolated midline spikes, polyspikes, or pathological sharp waves are most often noted at the central vertex, and have a high association with epilepsy. No distinct clinical syndrome exists for patients with midline spikes. Tonic seizures are the most frequent clinical seizure type that is associated with midline IEDs. Midline EEG electrodes with vertex representation are important to detect discharges in this region.

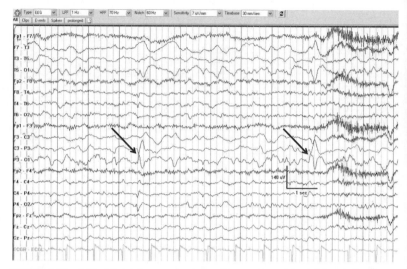

FIGURE 3.11. Left parietal sharp waves (arrows) in a patient with a left hemispheric stroke requiring resuscitation. Note the continuous left hemispheric slowing that is also present.

In patients with parietal lobe epilepsy, the scalp EEG is often of limited yield. Pz spikes are rarely seen and when parietal IEDs occur they often appear (similar to FLE) as a secondary bilaterally synchronous discharge. The IEDs in this region may be falsely localizing or even falsely lateralizing. Centro-parietal spike ("CP spikes") may be noted in patients with a perinatal motor deficit without the presence of clinical seizures.

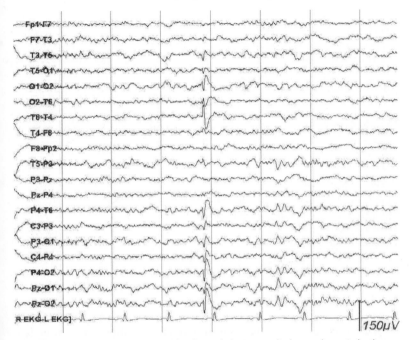

FIGURE 3.12. A single right occipital spike-and-slow wave discharge shown in both a bipolar and reference montage (last two channels).

Occipital IEDs are most frequently reported in the benign childhood epilepsies with occipital paroxysms and the later-onset Panayioto-poulos syndrome. Occipital spikes are infrequently localized to a single occipital lobe (above) and are more likely to appear bilateral. They may also falsely localize and often do so in the temporal region. Occipital IEDs may also appear in nonepileptic patients who express the IEDs as a genetic trait, or appear in patients who are congenitally blind ("needle spikes" of the blind). Occipital IEDs have been noted in children with visual dysfunction, the benign occipital epilepsies of childhood, and also in adults with structural lesions and symptomatic occipital lobe epilepsy with or without a visual aura.

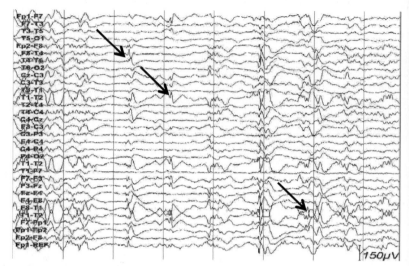

FIGURE 3.13. Multifocal independent spike discharges (arrows) in a patient with mental retardation and drug-resistant encephalopathic generalized epilepsy.

Multifocal spikes may be seen in individuals with discrete structural lesions, although usually they are associated with diffuse structural injury involving the gray matter of the hemispheres. Mental retardation and cerebral palsy are common underlying substrates for patients with multifocal independent spike discharges. There may be a primary site of focal dysfunction or be associated with concomitant generalized epileptiform discharges that are not uncommonly seen in patients with the Lennox-Gastaut syndrome (LGS).

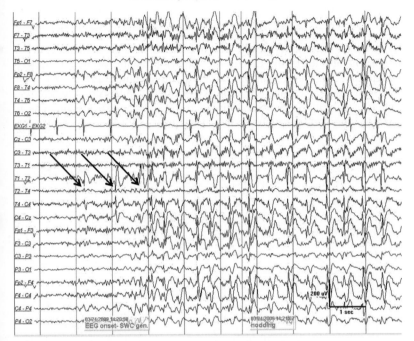

FIGURE 3.14. A secondary bilateral synchronous (SBS) burst of sharp-and-slow waves. Note the right frontotemporal spikes 2 seconds prior to the burst (arrows).

SBS is a term used to refer to a generalized discharge with a focal onset. These diffuse bursts are best distinguished when a "lead in" of 400 msec or more is noted in a patient with independent focal IEDs. Patients with medial frontal seizures such as those with supplementary motor area, medial frontal convexity, or cingulate gyrus area involvement are most likely to manifest SBS. Due to the proximity of these sites to the corpus callosum, there is a propensity for rapid bihemispheric propagation from a focal source.

GENERALIZED EPILEPTIFORM DISCHARGES

Generalized IEDs are typically seen in patients with generalized epilepsy and are helpful to classify the genetic and symptomatic forms. Generalized epileptiform discharges vary in duration with a continuum that blurs the interictal and ictal transformation. Generalized epileptiform discharges may be seen with or without clinical signs or even appear less often as an isolated inherited trait without clinical seizures.

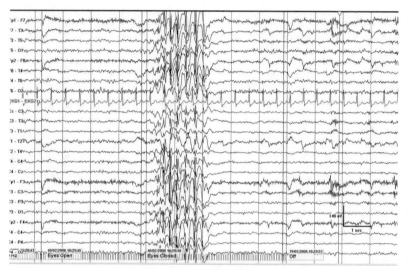

FIGURE 3.15. A self-limited photoparoxysmal response (PPR) during intermittent photic stimulation in a patient with a strong family history of seizures and migraine.

A PPR or photoconvulsive response consists of a burst of generalized epileptiform discharges typically consisting of spikes and/or poly-spike-and-slow wave (PSW) complexes that are provoked by photic stimulation. The most frequent provocative frequencies appear around 15 Hz. Eye closure may evoke the PPR and is typically performed during intermittent photic stimulation. It has a clinical correlation with photosensitivity and one of the genetic generalized epilepsies (GGEs), although it may also appear as an inherited trait without seizures (Figure 3.15). A non-self-limited PPR beyond the duration of the stimulus has been more frequently associated with epilepsy according to some investigators. Juvenile myoclonic epilepsy (JME), juvenile absence epilepsy, and childhood absence epilepsy in descending order of frequency may show photosensitivity.

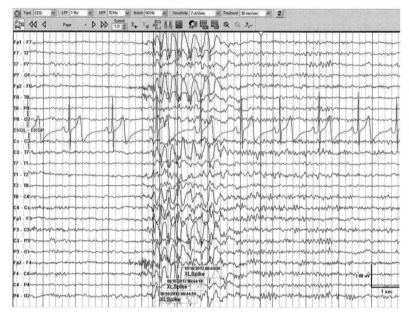

FIGURE 3.16. A burst of 3-4 Hz GSWs in a patient with juvenile absence epilepsy. The myogenic artifact immediately before suggests that the state change after represents an arousal response triggering an interictal burst (vs. a very brief absence seizure).

The prototypic abnormality on EEG seen with generalized seizures is the 3-Hz spike-and-slow-wave complex. It appears as a bilateral, synchronous, symmetrical, surface-negative spike maximal in the frontal-central regions, followed by a surface-negative slow wave in a longitudinal bipolar montage. Minor lateralized asymmetry may be observed. Response times may be impaired regardless of burst duration, although longer bursts imply a greater likelihood of impaired responsiveness. Alerting responses act to inhibit generalized spike-and-waves (GSW) discharges, while sleep, hyperventilation (HV), and intermittent photic stimulation often precipitate them in GGE. In sleep, the bursts of GSW may "fragment," and appear irregular and lateralized, have a slower repetition rate (less than 3 Hz), and have a greater predisposition to polyspike formation.

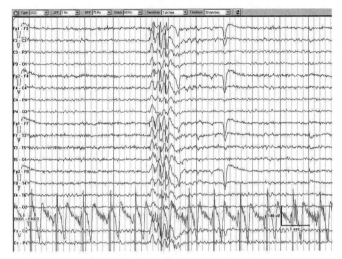

FIGURE 3.17A. A brief burst of 5 Hz generalized spike-and-slow-waves in a female patient with refractory myoclonus and JME.

Spike-and-slow-wave complexes that have a repetition rate of greater than 3 Hz are referred to as *fast GSW*. Juvenile myoclonic epilepsy (JME) is the most common idiopathic generalized epilepsy (IGE) syndrome associated with myoclonus and often demonstrates fast spike-and-slow wave complexes with frequencies of 3.5 to 5.0 Hz on the interictal EEG that may slow to 2.25 to 2.5 Hz during longer bursts. When "fast" GSW approaches a 6 Hz frequency normal variants ("phantom spike-and-wave) merit consideration. The high amplitude GSW in a female during sleep (Figure 3.17), the <6 Hz inter-spike frequency, and clinical history of myoclonic jerks help distinguish the abnormal discharge above. While generalized polyspike-and-slow-waves and "fast" GSW are most likely to occur in JME, the "typical" 3-Hz GSW may be seen in 25% of individuals. Lateralized features may also occur during seizures, as well as on EEG, although they probably represent fragmentation of the generalized discharge in the majority of cases.

(Continued)

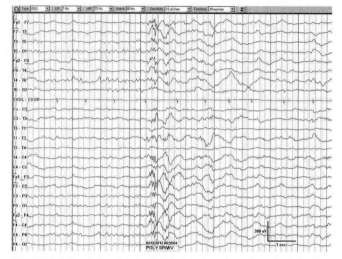

FIGURE 3.17B. Generalized polyspike-and-waves (PSW) during N1 sleep. Notice the series of slow waves that persists after the single polyspike.

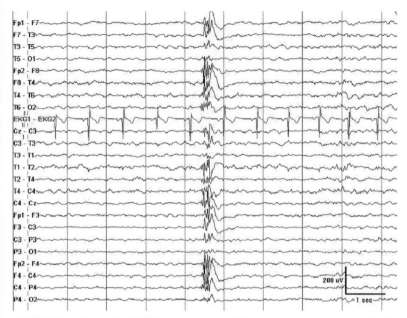

FIGURE 3.18. Generalized PSW in a patient with JME with myoclonus and generalized tonic-clonic seizures successfully controlled by antiepileptic drugs.

The most characteristic feature on EEG in patients with JME is generalized, bisynchronous, frontocentrally-predominant "fast" PSW complexes, although this may also be seen in other GGEs as well. The discharges are maximal in the frontal regions with two or more high-voltage surface-negative spikes best described as polyspikes (or multispikes). The incidence of the PSW bursts increases on transitioning to the awake state and frequently translates clinically to early morning myoclonus and GTC seizures. Sleep deprivation is a potent activator of the generalized IEDs seen with JME. Photosensitivity may occur in up to 40% of patients with JME and is more prominent in females.

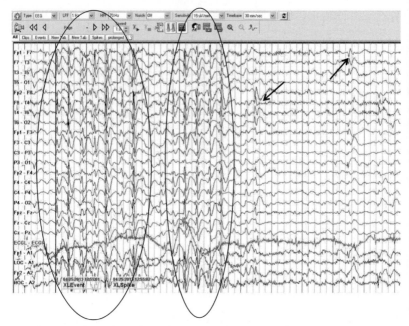

FIGURE 3.19. Slow spike-and-wave bursts (ovals) in a patient with Lennox-Gastaut syndrome. Note the diffusely slow background activity and independent spikes (arrows).

Slow spike(or sharp)-and-wave (SSW) discharges are generalized epileptiform discharges with a repetition rate of less than 3 Hz. They typically occur in patients with diffuse brain structural injury or dysfunction. SSW is one of the characteristic features on EEG of the Lennox-Gastaut syndrome (LGS). Many patients with West syndrome and hypsarhythmia evolve into the pattern of diffuse slowing, multifocal IEDs, and slow spike-and-waves characteristic of the LGS (see Figure 3.19). SSW may consist of a biphasic or triphasic surface negative sharp and slow wave complexes in a bilateral, synchronous, symmetrical, frontocentral burst. They often appear as repetitive bursts or runs of frequencies ranging from 1.5 to 2.5 Hz and are often asymmetrical or shifting, becoming prolonged runs during sleep. These IEDs are not activated with either HV or IPSP. A less discrete onset and offset with a longer duration is seen with the SSW discharges as opposed to that seen with "typical" 3-Hz GSW discharges. Most SSW bursts are interictal, although atypical absence seizures are the most common clinical ictal correlate.

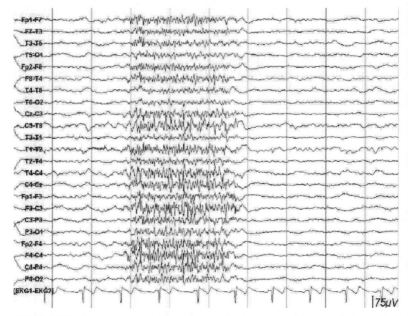

FIGURE 3.20. An asymptomatic burst of generalized paroxysmal fast activity in a patient with the Lennox-Gastaut syndrome and tonic seizures. The clinical presence of subtle tonic stiffening can often be verified with the use of electromyography though this has limited utility in the overall treatment.

Generalized paroxysmal fast activity (GPFA) is another "interictal epileptiform discharge" on the EEG that often occurs with the SSW and multi-focal independent spike discharges of LGS. It is primarily seen during sleep and consists of sudden, discrete, diffuse of bilateral 15 to 20 Hz frontally predominant fast activity. Variable frequencies, voltages, and durations may occur, although they usually last several seconds and appear as generalized polyspike discharges when brief. This feature frequently has no overtly detectable clinical manifestations, although it may correlate with tonic seizures when occurring while awake or with durations of greater than 6 seconds.

ADDITIONAL RESOURCES

Abraham K, Ajmone-Marsan C. Patterns of cortical discharges and their relation to routine scalp electroencephalography. *Electroencephalogr Clin Neurophysiol Suppl.* 1958;10:447-461.

Ebersole JS. Defining epileptogenic foci: past, present, and future. *J Clin Neurophysiol.* 1997;14:470-483.

Gregory RP, Oates T, Merry RT. Electroencephalogram epileptiform abnormalities in candidates for aircrew training. *Electroencephalogr Clin Neurophysiol.* 1993;86:75-77.

Maulsby RL. Some guidelines for the assessment of spikes and sharp waves in EEG tracings. *Am J EEG Technol.* 1971;11:3-16.

Pedley TA, Mendiratta A, Walczak TS. Seizures and epilepsy. In: Ebersole JS, Pedley TA, eds. *Current Practice of Clinical Electroencephalography.* 3rd ed. Philadelphia, PA: Lippincott Williams & Wilkins; 2003:506-587.

Pillai J, Sperling MR. Interictal EEG and the diagnosis of epilepsy. *Epilepsia.* 2006;47(suppl 1):14-22.

Shewmon DA, Erwin RJ. The effect of focal interictal spikes on perception of reaction time. I. General considerations. *Electroencephalogr Clin Neurophysiol.* 1988;69:319-377.

So EL. Interictal epileptiform discharges in persons without a history of seizures: what do they mean? *J Clin Neurophysiol.* 2010;27:229-238.

Tao JX, Ray A, Hawes-Ebersole S, Ebersole JS. Intracranial EEG substrates of scalp EEG interictal spikes. *Epilepsia.* 2005;46(5):669-676.

Westmoreland B. Epileptiform electroencephalographic patterns. *Mayo Clin Proc.* 1996;71:501-511.

Zifkin BG. The electroencephalogram as a screening tool in pilot applicants. *Epilepsy Behav.* 2005;6:17-20.

4

Pediatric Seizures

Douglas R. Nordli, Jr

The typical convention is to divide seizures into either focal or generalized types based largely upon the accompanying EEG ictal patterns. In the most recent publication from the International League Against Epilepsy (ILAE) this tradition was continued and recognizes generalized, focal, and unknown seizure types. All of these seizure types are seen in children (Table 4.1). The generalized seizures are easily recognized by their descriptive titles. There is also widespread agreement and ease with their use. The classification of focal seizures is another matter, and to some extent remains a work in progress. One popular method is to base the classification upon descriptive terms, according to the semiology of the seizures. This approach works well and is very amenable to young children. It complements the semiological descriptions recommended by some authors for neonates and infants which will be briefly reviewed here. Finally, only one seizure is currently listed in the "unknown" category and that is epileptic spasms, of which infantile spasms (IS) is the most well-known subtype.

TABLE 4.1. Generalized Seizures

Tonic-clonic (in any combination)

Absence

  Typical

  Atypical

  Absence with special features

    Myoclonic absence

    Eyelid myoclonia

Myoclonic

  Myoclonic

  Myoclonic atonic

  Myoclonic tonic

Clonic

Tonic

Atonic

Focal seizures

Unknown

  Epileptic spasms

GENERALIZED SEIZURES

Generalized tonic-clonic (GTC) seizures can be seen at nearly any age, but are rarely seen in infancy. In the Genetic Generalized Epilepsies (GGEs) these seizures often begin with brief clonic jerking or a few myoclonic jerks that are rapidly followed by the stiffening phase (tonic) and culminating in the rhythmic jerking phase (clonic). The earliest manifestation is often eye opening, often with upward deviation of the eyes. The tonic phase is caused by sustained contractions of the muscles, often lasting 10 to 20 seconds. A wide variety of postures may be seen in this phase, but many times the arms are flexed at the elbows while the legs are fully extended. A forced exhalation at this stage can produce a loud noise that alerts parents to the presence of the seizure. Repeated jerking of the limbs characterizes the clonic portion of the seizure which often lasts 30 seconds to a minute. There may be accompanying bladder or bowel incontinence and tongue biting can occur. Afterwards, the child is temporarily comatose. Breathing resumes with a deep breath and the child gradually returns to normal function after a variable postictal phase.

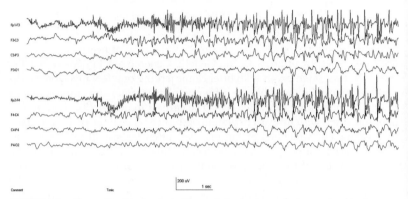

FIGURE 4.1. Generalized tonic-clonic. The early tonic phase of a generalized tonic-clonic seizure is shown from the recording done on a 25 year-old.

The ictal EEG often begins with diffuse spikes, correlating with the brief clonic or myoclonic onset. The tonic phase may begin with a brief epoch of diffuse flattening (Figure 4.1), followed by diffuse rhythmic low voltage beta activity, and finally a sustained 10 to 12 Hz rhythm (epileptic recruiting rhythm).

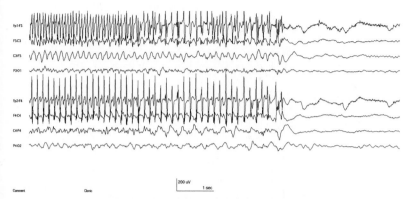

FIGURE 4.2. Generalized tonic-clonic. The clonic phase of a generalized tonic-clonic seizure is shown from the same child in Figure 4.1.

During the clonic phase, there are repeated bursts of high amplitude spike or polyspike-wave complexes correlating with the individual jerks (Figure 4.2). In the postictal period, there is either profound background suppression or diffuse background slowing. The polygraphic recording will show a rectangular shape in the tonic phase of the seizure. This is due to the abundant, very fast reciprocal tonic contractions of the muscles. This is followed by rhythmic contractions during the clonic phase. In the immediate postictal epoch the muscle tone will be very low and the polygraphic channels will be flat.

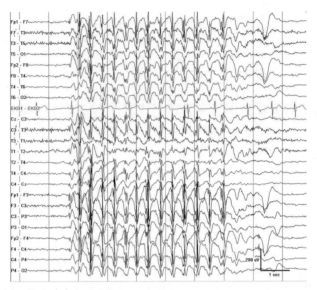

FIGURE 4.3. Typical absence seizure.

Typical and atypical absence seizures are most easily distinguished by characteristics defined by their EEG. Typical absence seizures have a faster repetition rate (3–4 Hz), whereas the ictal accompaniment of atypical absences seizures has a repetition rate less than or equal to 2.5 Hz. Atypical absence seizures have an indiscrete onset and offset and are more prolonged than typical absence seizures. Atypical absence seizures typically occur in the encephalopathic generalized epilepsies.

In contrast, typical absence seizures are brief events with a very distinct start and finish. There are two required features: there is some impairment in consciousness with the seizure and the EEG demonstrates bursts of generalized 3 to 4 Hz spike-and-wave activity (Figure 4.3). Some experts further divide typical absence seizures into simple and complex categories, depending on the presence (complex) or lack (simple) of motor features. The latest publication from the ILAE describes two types of absence seizures with special features: so-called myoclonic absence and absence with eyelid myoclonia.

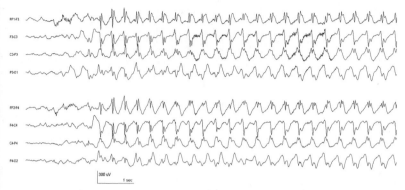

FIGURE 4.4. Absence. This 6 year-old was unresponsive during this burst of generalized 3 Hz spike-wave activity.

In typical absence seizures, children will usually develop an abrupt change in the countenance, a behavioral pause, and exhibit a stare. There is accompanying 3 to 4 Hz generalized spike-and-wave activity on the EEG (Figure 4.4). Importantly, the child must manifest some impairment of consciousness in order to declare the event a seizure because EEG bursts of generalized spike-wave discharges can occur without any symptoms. Most pediatric absence seizures will also show some motor manifestations such as jerks of the eyes, face, and body although they may be quite subtle. Oral automatisms may additionally be present.

The classic highly rhythmic 3 Hz spike-and-wave ictal discharge is often preceded by a short epoch of rhythmic slowing which may not be perfectly generalized. Instead, it may predominate posteriorly or anteriorly and contain admixed spikes. These bursts may be fragmented and not appear to be symmetrical. The initial phase usually lasts just a second or two and then the regular spike-and-wave discharges develop, entrained with the preceding rhythmic activity. There may be one or two spikes per spike-wave complex, but three spikes per complex denotes polyspike-and-wave activity. Absence seizures begin with repetitive generalized spike-and-wave discharges that typically last 5 to 10 seconds. During the terminal phase of the seizure, rhythmic slowing occurs with fragmented spikes as the EEG rapidly recovers to baseline.

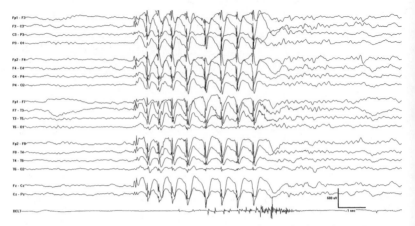

FIGURE 4.5. Myoclonic absence. Note the presence of several jerks in the EMG channel accompanying this burst of generalized spike-wave activity.

Myoclonic absence is a rare variant of absence with special features. Although it is described as a myoclonic absence seizure, they actually begin with a sudden tonic elevation of the arms followed by brief clonic activity. With each jerk the arms may raise further as the body slumps forward. The ictal pattern is characterized by a typical absence pattern with generalized 3 Hz spike-wave discharges (Figure 4.5).

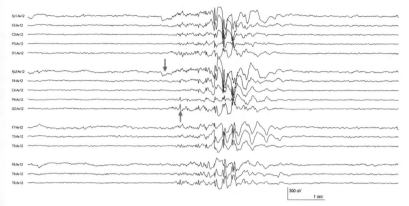

FIGURE 4.6. Eyelid Myoclonia. This 12-year-old had eye fluttering after eye closure. Note the eye closure artifact (top arrow), followed moments later by the rhythmic occipital discharge (bottom arrow).

Aunique type of seizure that is often classified with absence seizures is absence with eyelid myoclonia. It is the principal seizure seen in Jeavons syndrome, but it is also seen in other conditions, including Dravet syndrome. During these seizures there is, as the name suggests, prominent eyelid myoclonia composed of fast eyelid fluttering. A peculiar feature of these seizures is that these ictal discharges often follow slow eye closure to provide an unmistakable and characteristic electroclinical syndrome. The EEG pattern that follows the slow eye closure occurs in less than one second. It is comprised of a build-up of rhythmic fast activity in the posterior quadrants that leads to more diffuse spike- or polyspike-and-wave discharges (Figure 4.6). The total duration is often brief, lasting a few seconds or so, and the baseline activity then rapidly returns. There may be an alteration of consciousness during the event, but this is not invariable even during the eyelid myoclonia. Therefore, some regard this as a myoclonic seizure more so than an absence seizure.

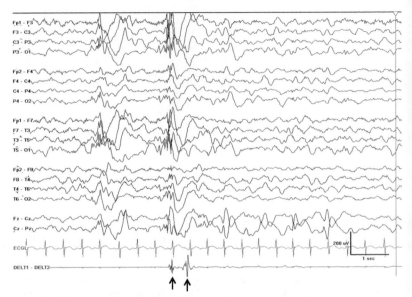

FIGURE 4.7. Myoclonic. A myoclonic seizure is shown and this is often accompanied by a burst of generalized spike-wave activity. Note the myogenic artifact in the deltoid surface EMG (arrows) produced by the myoclonic jerk.

Myoclonic seizures are very brief contractures of the muscles causing a abrupt lighting fast jerk. They may involve just about any part or segment of the body, or can involve the entire body. On EEG the jerk is usually time locked to a burst of diffuse polyspike-and-wave activity. Sometimes an electrodecrement in background activity may occur in association with the myoclonus (Figure 4.7). The polygraphic channels will show a sudden burst of muscle activity, usually lasting less than 100 msec.

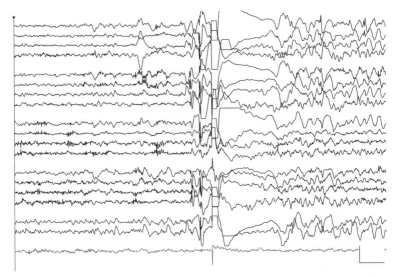

FIGURE 4.8. Myoclonic-atonic. A myoclonic-atonic seizure was recorded in a 6-year-old.

Myoclonic-atonic seizures were formerly known as myoclonic-astatic seizures. They are another important seizure type to recognize because they are an indispensible cornerstone for the diagnosis of Doose syndrome. This is mostly seen in childhood. There is a sudden myoclonic component that often causes the arms to jerk and this is followed by a sudden diffuse loss of muscle tone. This loss of tone can result in just a head nod, a collapse of the upper body tone, or of the entire body. In the more severe cases myoclonic absences result in an abrupt fall which may lead to injury due to the sudden and unpredictable nature of the events. The morbidity that results may include lacerations of the head and face, dislodged teeth, fractured bones, burns and serious injuries. The myoclonic portion of the seizure is accompanied by a diffuse polyspike discharge and the atonic portion correlates with a diffuse decrement (Figure 4.8). Polygraphic tracings with deltoid electromyography (EMG) recordings are very helpful in supporting the diagnosis. There is evidence of accompanying brief muscle contraction followed by a sudden loss of tone.

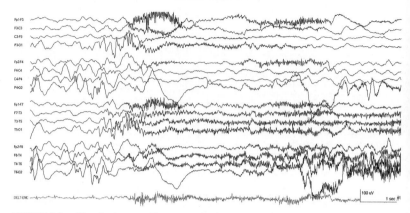

FIGURE 4.9. Myoclonic-tonic. This 5-month-old had a sudden jerk followed by diffuse stiffening. Note the electrodecremental response followed by the rhythmic fast activity.

Myoclonic-tonic seizures may be seen across the pediatric age span, but are most commonly observed in infants and young children (Figure 5.6). They are a common seizure type seen in infants with severe epileptic encephalopathies over 1 year of age. As the name suggests, the seizure begins with a rapid jerk. This can involve multiple regions of the body, but it often is prominently seen in the child's arms. This is rapidly followed by stiffening of the skeletal musculature lasting several seconds. On EEG, these seizures begin with an electrodecrement and are followed by runs of diffuse fast activity (Figure 4.9). The polygraphic channels that record surface EMG show the typical pattern of rapid and brief muscular activity during the myoclonic component and sustained very fast rhythmic activity resembling a rectangular shape during the tonic phase. Spasm-tonic seizures are probably a closely related (or identical) phenomenon where the initial movement on video and polygraphic tracings appears to last longer than a typical myoclonic jerk.

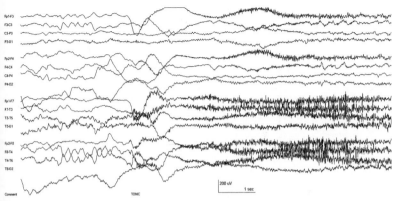

FIGURE 4.10. Tonic. This was a recording done on an 8-month-old with a tonic seizure. Note the low voltage fast activity diffusely.

Generalized clonic seizures are rarely seen outside of the early infantile period. Rhythmic jerking of the arms, legs, or both is seen at the onset without any pronounced focal signature. The ictal EEG correlate is a run of synchronous spike-wave activity that is often maximal in the rolandic region.

Generalized tonic seizures involve some form of sustained stiffening of the skeletal musculature. They may vary in the degree and somatic distribution of involvement. Gastaut and colleagues described three different types. Tonic seizures may be *axial* seizures consisting of eye opening with stiffening of the paraspinal musculature. In *axorhizomelic* seizures, the proximal portion of the arms and legs are involved. The most florid manifestations are *global* where the entire body stiffens. The commonest EEG accompaniment is a paroxysmal discharge composed of diffuse low voltage fast activity (Figure 4.10).

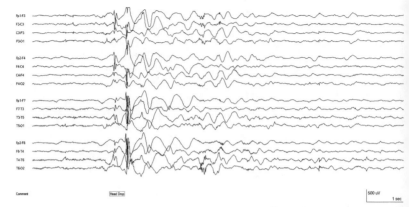

FIGURE 4.11. Atonic. A sudden head drop was the correlate of these diffuse spike-wave discharges in a 4-year-old.

Atonic seizures involve a sudden loss of tone. This may affect only a specific portion of the body such as the neck musculature, a larger segment such as the upper torso, or the body more diffusely. The ictal EEG correlate is usually an electrodecrement, but may also be a burst of spike- or polyspike-and-wave activity (Figure 4.11).

FOCAL SEIZURES

It is very difficult or sometime impossible to accurately determine alteration of consciousness during a seizure in very young patients. Certainly, for preverbal infants, or children with special needs, it may be entirely out of the question. Even in the slightly older, preschool population, this task may be daunting. For that reason the standard simple versus complex differential cannot be reliably applied to many pediatric seizures. Young children also do not volunteer eloquent descriptions of the ictal sensations, and perhaps it is not possible to declare auras before one has developed a repertoire of experiential memories. Lastly, there are profound differences in the motor manifestations of focal seizures in the immature which limit the ability to precisely localize the seizures. Taking all of these factors into consideration, a simple, practical, and semiological classification can be fashioned and used reliably in the very young. In older children and adults it is very helpful to link together various semiological features such as the classification system developed by Lüders and colleagues. However, in the immature, brain seizures have less secondary generalization during early development, so in this age group the following terminology may be used to characterize seizures.

Asymmetric epileptic spasms, as well as focal clonic, myoclonic, and tonic seizures, have similar EEG characteristics and parameters to their generalized counterparts, except that the EEG patterns are restricted to one region or side of the brain.

TABLE 4.2. Common Focal Seizures in the Very Young

Behavioral arrest (hypomotor)
Clonic (face, arm, leg, or combination)
Epileptic spasms (asymmetric variety)
Myoclonic (focal as opposed to generalized)
Tonic (focal as opposed to generalized)
Versive (eyes, head, or both)

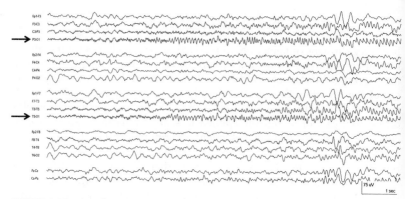

FIGURE 4.12. Focal. Focal seizures often have a crescendo pattern like this one seen from the left occipital region (arrows).

Most focal seizures begin with focal or regional rhythmic activities that slow in frequency as they build in amplitude. As they evolve they propagate to adjacent brain regions. The net result of this is to create an appearance on EEG like a crescendo mark in music (Figure 4.12). Behavioral arrest and versive seizures are clinical features that are commonly seen when seizures arise from the temporal lobe or posterior quadrant. Focal clonic seizures often arise from the central region. Tonic seizures may have an origin from nearly any region in the brain, but commonly the frontal lobe. Overall, there is less secondary generalization in seizures of the very young. In addition, the seizures do not include auras, automatisms, or dystonic postures.

UNKNOWN ORIGIN

Epileptic Spasms

Infantile Spasms

Epileptic spasm is a term used to broadly cover all of the different types of spasms recorded throughout the age spectrum. Infantile spasms (IS) are one important subgroup that are usually manifest in the first year of life. IS are composed of clusters of individual spasms separated by 5 to 10 second intervals. Usually the spacing between the individual spasms is fairly regular, although there may be variation during a cluster. The entire cluster itself can last many minutes in duration. There is a tendency for the clusters to occur upon awakening, or just upon going to sleep. The spasm starts with a sudden jolt affecting the head, limbs, torso, or the entire body. Simultaneous upward eye deviation (sursum vergens) is sometimes the subtlest but earliest feature of IS. The neck may flex and then the trunk may flex with extension of the arms. The presentation resembles the salaam greeting reflected in the German description: blitz-nick-salaam for the sequence of IS. Variations on this theme are common with flexion instead of extension, or mixtures of flexion/extension movements. The entire spasm usually lasts less than a second. It has a diamond or rhomboid shape that appears on the polygraphic channel.

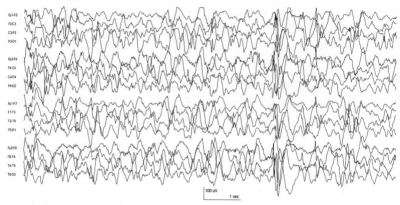

FIGURE 4.13. Hypsarhythmia. This 9-month-old presents with infantile spasms. The EEG is high voltage and chaotic. There are superimposed multifocal spikes.

The classic interictal EEG finding is hypsarhythmia—a high voltage (greater than 300 μV) disorganized background with superimposed multifocal spikes and epochs of discontinuity (Figure 4.13). This classic pattern does not occur in all babies, and in fact, may only be seen in about 60% of the initial recordings. Jeavons and Bower found that nearly all EEGs will be abnormal at presentation, but not necessarily as profoundly abnormal as the hypsarhythmia pattern. (The term hypsarhythmia was coined by Gibbs and one "r" is used in the text to honor their original description).

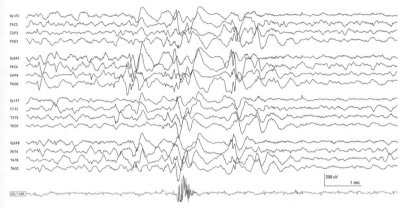

FIGURE 4.14. Electrodecremental response. The EEG correlate of a spasm is an electrodecremental response, shown here in a 9-month-old.

The ictal EEG correlate is called an electrodecrement (Figure 4.14). It is a complex discharge and may involve one or several features. First and most consistently there is a high voltage slow wave transient that is maximal at the vertex. Second, there are often admixed multifocal spikes embedded in the high voltage slow wave transient. Third, there is a diffuse and abrupt attenuation of the entire EEG lasting one to several seconds. Fourth, and last, there may be admixed low voltage fast activity embedded in the otherwise diffusely attenuated background. In the experience of the author (DN), this low voltage fast is not a reliable indicator of focal cortical pathology.

Periodic Spasms

Periodic spasms are another form of epileptic spasms. They typically occur outside of the infantile period. They are superimposed on a normal EEG background. As the name suggests, they have a very regular interval between each individual epileptic spasm and typically cluster for several minutes.

Other Epileptic Spasms

Epileptic spasms may be seen in early infancy in a variety of epileptic encephalopathies, including that described by Ohtahara. They may consist of isolated spasms, though are sometimes associated with other seizure types like tonic seizures and myoclonia. In our epilepsy monitoring unit, epileptic spasms occur twice as commonly outside of infancy as they do in infancy. They may appear after other seizures, for example, following tonic seizures in patients with Lennox-Gastaut syndrome. In later infancy they blend together with myoclonic-tonic seizures (in Late Infantile Epileptic Encephalopathy), and sometimes are referred to as late onset epileptic spasms or spasm-tonic seizures.

FINAL COMMENTS

The astute reader may have noticed that there are only a few different types of ictal patterns on EEG. The commonest correlate of a focal seizure is the crescendo pattern which begins with a focal run of rhythmic activity. Absence, atypical absence, myoclonic seizures, and some atonic seizures all have bursts of generalized spike-and-wave discharges. Epileptic spasms, myoclonic-tonic, and some atonic seizures usually have electrodecremental correlates on ictal EEG. Most tonic seizures are associated with a diffuse low voltage rhythmic fast discharge. The polygraphic channels are very helpful to get a quick sense of the clinical correlate. The ictal discharge on EEG is better characterized by measuring motor patterns of the seizure. Generalized seizures have descriptive names that nicely sum up their principle features. Focal seizures require a more elaborate description based upon their semiology. In adults, the clinical features can be very localizing, but this is infrequently the case in the very young patient, though progressively become more useful as patients approach 5 to 6 years of age.

ADDITIONAL RESOURCES

Berg AT, Berkovic SF, Brodie MJ, et al. Revised terminology and concepts for organization of seizures and epilepsies: report of the ILAE Commission on Classification and Terminology, 2005-2009. *Epilepsia*. 2010;51:676-685.

Bower BD, Jeavons PM. Infantile spasms and hypsarrhythmia. *Lancet*. 1959; 1:605-609.

Fusco L, Vigevano F. Ictal clinical electroencephalographic findings of spasms in West syndrome. *Epilepsia*. 1993;34:671-678.

Gastaut H, Roger J, Ouahchi S, Timsit M, Broughton R. An electro-clinical study of generalized epileptic seizures of tonic expression. *Epilepsia*. 1963;4:15-44.

Gibbs EL, Fleming MM, Gibbs FA. Diagnosis and prognosis of hypsarhythmia and infantile spasms. *Pediatrics*. 1954;13:66-73.

Korff C, Nordli DR, Jr. Do generalized tonic-clonic seizures in infancy exist? *Neurology*. 2005;65:1750-1753.

Luders H, Acharya J, Baumgartner C, et al. Semiological seizure classification. *Epilepsia*. 1998;39:1006-1013.

Nordli DR, Jr, Bazil CW, Scheuer ML, Pedley TA. Recognition and classification of seizures in infants. *Epilepsia*. 1997;38:553-560.

Stephani U. The natural history of myoclonic astatic epilepsy (Doose syndrome) and Lennox-Gastaut syndrome. *Epilepsia*. 2006;47(suppl 2):53-55.

Viravan S, Go C, Ochi A, Akiyama T, Carter Snead O, 3rd, Otsubo H. Jeavons syndrome existing as occipital cortex initiating generalized epilepsy. *Epilepsia*. 2011;52:1273-1279.

Volpe JJ. Neonatal seizures: current concepts and revised classification. *Pediatrics*. 1989;84:422-428.

5

Adult Seizures

William O. Tatum, IV and
Peter W. Kaplan

The EEG is able to provide a definitive diagnosis of epilepsy when seizures are recorded. Additionally, classifying the seizure type and characterizing the localization of recurrent seizures in epilepsy may be useful not only in the diagnosis, but also in the treatment selection and prognosis. The EEG provides only supportive information for the clinical diagnosis of epilepsy when interictal epileptiform discharges (IEDs) are present because, unless a seizure is recorded, IEDs may appear and be unassociated with clinical seizures. In pediatric patients, generalized seizures are common, while in the adult focal seizures predominate. Generalized onset seizures are more stereotyped than focal seizures. For focal seizures, there are a wide variety of paroxysmal EEG patterns that express a change in frequency, amplitude, distribution, and rhythmicity of the evolving ictal discharge. The EEG during seizures is most frequently composed of evolving sustained rhythmic frequencies as opposed to simple repetition of the interictal IEDs. There is an interictal-ictal spectrum of activity on the EEG that is best served when defined as a continuum. Furthermore, the EEG may indicate electrographic evidence of seizures even in the absence of a clinical correlate. Seizures may be evident on the EEG in cases of altered mental status or cognitive awareness, especially when the seizures that occur are nonconvulsive and are not overtly visible to others. Monitoring the EEG in the intensive care unit, critical care unit, or emergency department may provide diagnostic input that affects the clinical approach to treatment when seizures or status epilepticus is encountered. This chapter will provide the seizure types and their associated EEG findings.

CHAPTER 5

GENERALIZED SEIZURES

Generalized seizures have a greater homogeneous semiology compared to focal seizures. In genetic generalized epilepsy, several seizure types may coexist and overlap in different epilepsy syndromes despite a common ictal EEG pattern. Generalized seizures associated with encephalopathic generalized epilepsy are more heterogeneous due to the variety of symptomatic etiologies that can occur, but have the common characteristic of an underlying diffuse structural injury of the brain.

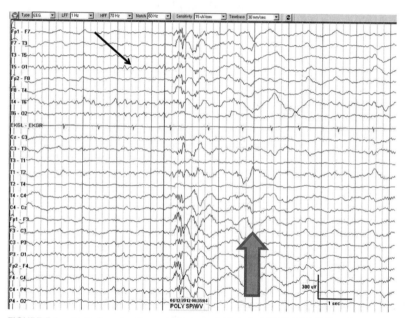

FIGURE 5.1. A single polyspike and slow-wave(s) (labeled "POLY SP/WV") with subsequent "slowing" (big arrow) noted in the background and state change. Note the POSTS (thin arrow) in N1 sleep prior to the "interictal" epileptiform discharge.

(Continued)

Most generalized spike-and-wave discharges that are shorter than 3 sec in duration *do not* typically demonstrate clinically noticeable signs. However, even a single spike-and-wave discharge may be associated with a subtle behavioral alteration of responsiveness that is not clinically apparent using gross testing modalities. Notice the above "post-ictal" slowing following a single generalized polyspike-and-slow wave discharge. Even a single discharge may be associated with a change in the level of alertness felt to be potentially responsible for transient cognitive impairment.

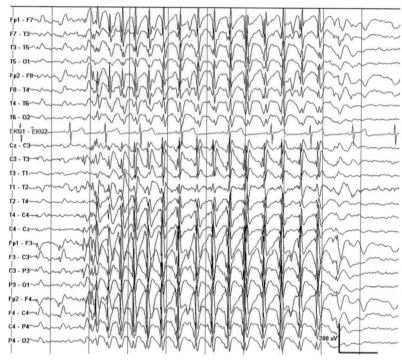

FIGURE 5.2. Absence seizure in an adult with juvenile absence epilepsy and absence, generalized tonic-clonic, and rare myoclonic seizures. Note the polyspike onset and the evolution to a 2 Hz frequency at seizure termination.

The 3-Hz spike-and-wave pattern is suggestive of genetic generalized epilepsy. When bursts of 3-Hz spike-and-waves are generalized, regular, symmetrical, synchronous, and maximal in the anterior head regions and are longer than 3 sec, the EEG strongly suggests the diagnosis of absence seizures (petit mal) though this pattern may be an ictal pattern seen with other seizure types (see above). During sleep, absence seizures may become more irregular and longer in duration. In addition, like the seizure semiology, the EEG may show asymmetries or lateralizing features during absence seizures. In adulthood, focal discharges have been seen following absence seizures rarely. With advancing age, absence seizures become more irregular and slow in the frequency of the repetition rate to less than 3 Hz.

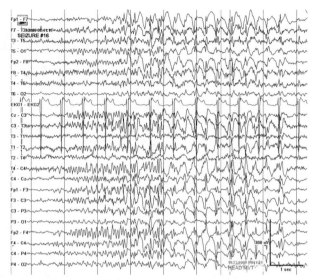

FIGURE 5.3. An atypical absence seizure in an adult with encephalopathic refractory generalized epilepsy. Notice the initial burst of generalized polyspikes that evolves to a 2.0–3.0 Hz spike-and-wave pattern.

Atypical absence seizures are clinically similar to typical absence seizures (Figure 5.3 and Chapter 4) however, during an atypical absence seizure, patients may have more incomplete loss of awareness and responsiveness. On the EEG, the bursts and IEDs often have a more gradual onset and offset and may be longer in duration. Slow spike-and-wave bursts accompany atypical absence seizures and have an inter-spike interval of less than 2.5-Hz frequency in the awake state. They may also have sharp waves or polyspikes prior to or intermixed with the aftergoing slow waves in the bursts (see above). There are frequent asymmetries and they are often associated with patients that have epilepsy with multifocal IEDs.

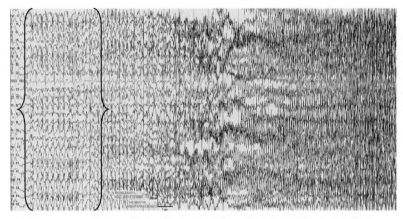

FIGURE 5.4. Myoclonic jerks (brackets) were followed by a generalized tonic-clonic seizure in a patient with clonic-tonic-clonic seizures associated with the JME syndrome.

Myoclonic seizures may be associated with a single complex (Figure 5.1) or burst of generalized spike or polyspike-and-waves (see above). Isolated polyspike-and-wave discharges may be associated with myoclonus that obscures the IED due to the overriding myogenic artifact created by the myoclonus. Fast visual display speeds and extracerebral electrodes may become helpful to distinguish myogenic spikes from that of polyspikes of cerebral origin. The polyspike formation was evident in the example above at the onset of the generalized seizure associated with myoclonus.

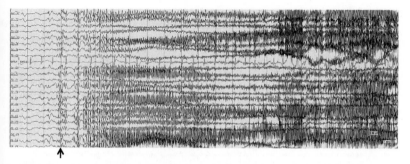

FIGURE 5.5. This EEG represented a tonic-clonic seizure in a patient with genetic generalized epilepsy manifest as recurrent generalized tonic-clonic seizures on awakening. Note the evolution from single epileptiform complexes (arrow) to continuous myogenic artifact.

Generalized tonic-clonic (GTC), or "grand mal" seizures, are often the most dramatic of the generalized seizures with a motor tonic and clonic component. The EEG demonstrates a "recruiting rhythm" that is composed of repetitive alpha frequencies in the maximal anterior head regions. Myogenic artifact subsequently obscures the record prior to the decrescendo phasic movement artifact from the clonic phase of the seizure that gradually stops prior to postictal suppression seen on the EEG. The GTC seizure may be seen in genetic generalized epilepsy without a focal origin, or generalize rapidly following a focal onset seizure. Lateralized and focal features suggest the latter situation where generalized motor seizures have a focal onset.

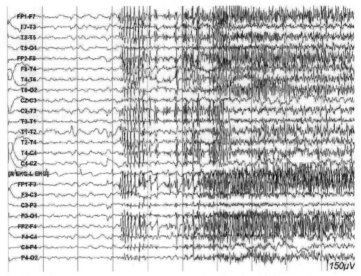

FIGURE 5.6. Tonic seizure in a patient with Lennox-Gastaut syndrome.

Tonic seizures are associated with symptomatic generalized epilepsy and are the most common seizure type associated with the Lennox-Gastaut syndrome. Tonic seizures typically have an abrupt onset of a generalized 10-Hz rhythm on EEG. Generalized paroxysmal fast activity is often seen as the associated features on EEG, although it may have no apparent clinical features associated with brief bursts that occur during sleep. Low-voltage fast frequencies associated with a generalized attenuation of the background may also be evident during a tonic seizure.

FOCAL SEIZURES

Focal seizures are the most common seizure type seen in adults. The ictal EEG can demonstrate a wide variety of abnormalities. The pattern and complexity that occurs on scalp EEG is dependent upon the location of the epileptogenic zone generating the seizure. Some focal seizures have no detectable representation at the surface of the scalp recorded EEG when they arise from buried cortex or involve a small region of cortex. Furthermore, some focal seizures have an ictal EEG pattern that is diffuse and appear falsely "generalized" in distribution or even appear to be "subclinical" with subtle or without apparent clinical signs.

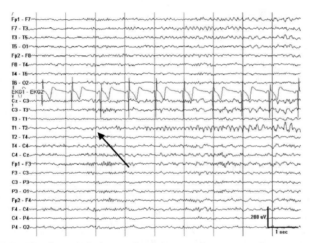

FIGURE 5.7. The above EEG shows a focal seizure without impaired consciousness that occurred out of N2 sleep (arrow).

Focal seizures that do not involve impairment of consciousness and are unassociated with clinical features reflect the aura. Most patients with mesial temporal lobe epilepsy (TLE) report an aura. However, while auras are nonspecific, experiential, or viscerosensory symptoms, including rising epigastric sensations, "butterflies," nausea, fear, and deja vu are common. Despite the presence of clinical symptoms, auras may be detected by scalp EEG only approximately 30% to 40% of the time on routine scalp EEG recording.

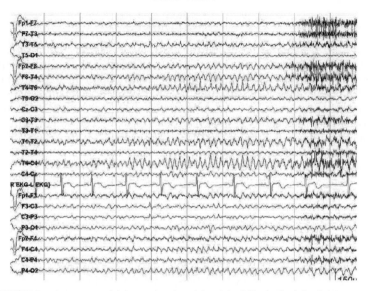

FIGURE 5.8. A paroxysmal right temporal evolving 6- to 7-Hz rhythmic ictal theta pattern on EEG at seizure onset in a patient with right mesial TLE.

Mesial temporal lobe seizures are the most common adult seizure type. Most seizures are composed of focal seizure with dyscognitive features impairing consciousness. Interictal EEG manifestations include anterior temporal spikes that are maximal at T1/F7 and T2/F8. Focal slowing and temporal intermittent rhythmic 2 to 4 Hz may appear and be facilitated by drowsiness and light non-rapid eye movement (non-REM) sleep. A frequent ictal pattern of mesial temporal origin is the sudden appearance of localized or regional background attenuation, build-up of 4- to 9-Hz rhythmic ictal theta or alpha activity that increases in amplitude as it slows to 1 to 2 Hz. This may be followed by post-ictal focal or diffuse suppression or slow activity.

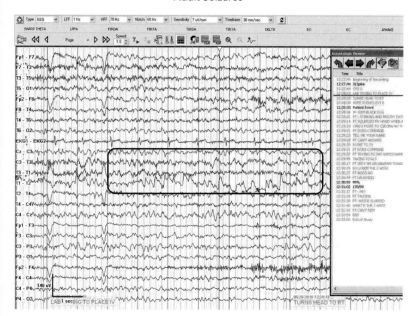

FIGURE 5.9. A left temporal neocortical seizure onset with subtle onset and irregular 3-Hz delta (box) that is maximal in the mid-temporal derivation prior to right head deviation and generalization.

Lateral or neocortical temporal seizures differ from those that begin in the mesial portion of the temporal lobe. Although it may be difficult to clinically distinguish neocortical temporal lobe seizures from mesial temporal lobe seizures, they often have a widespread hemispheric onset and begin in the mid-temporal derivations at less than 4 Hz. They typically have rapid propagation to the extratemporal neocortical structures and, therefore, have a greater likelihood to manifest a secondarily generalized motor seizure clinically with an ictal EEG as seen above. It is also not uncommon to have a bilateral ictal onset noted on EEG with neocortical temporal lobe seizure onset.

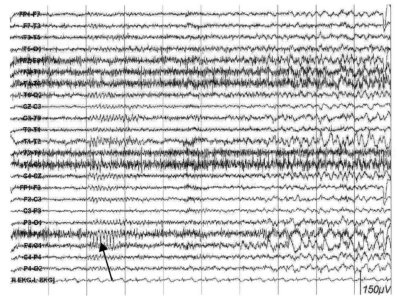

FIGURE 5.10. A temporal lobe seizure onset that falsely localizes to the right frontal region on scalp EEG. Note the initial burst of repetitive spiky alpha frequencies that evolve to the theta range.

Some patients with TLE may have projected rhythms to the anterior head regions often from the temporal pole. The reverse is also true in practice where 1/3rd of extratemporal seizure onset is noted to arise on scalp EEG in the temporal region. In the above example, a right anterior temporal lesion was present on high-resolution brain MRI and produced the appearance of an initial right frontal burst of repetitive spikes that evolved to an irregular right frontotemporal theta rhythm. The patient has been seizure free after right temporal lobectomy for greater than 2 years.

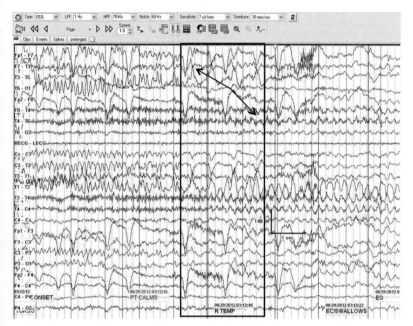

FIGURE 5.11. A left temporal lobe seizure onset "switching" to the right temporal region. Note the transitional period where both hemispheres "seize" at independent frequencies (rectangle).

Other patients with TLE may manifest a contralateral hemispheric propagation of the ictal activity after seizure onset. This suggests a tendency towards bihemispheric hyperexcitability and the possibility of more than one generator. The patient in Figure 5.11 demonstrated a "switch" from the left hemisphere to the right hemisphere and was ultimately proven to demonstrate an equal predisposition to bitemporal seizure onset determined by intracranial EEG. She was therefore felt to be a poor surgical candidate and was subsequently implanted with a responsive neurostimulator.

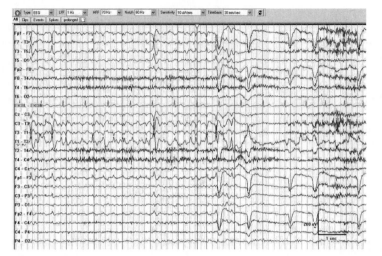

FIGURE 5.12. Generalized attenuation and loss of frequent interictal spiking in a patient with left posterior temporal neocortical epilepsy.

Some patients with TLE may manifest a loss of frequent interictal repetitive IEDs. These patients often have an extratemporal neocortical source for their seizure onset.

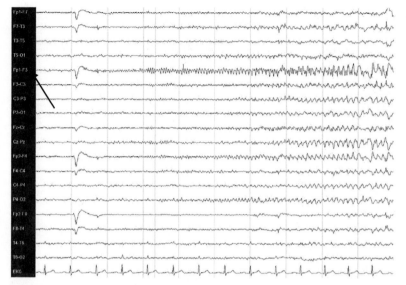

FIGURE 5.13. Discrete focal seizure onset (arrow) in a patient with a right frontal mass lesion. (Courtesy of Imran Ali, MD.). Note: this focal ictal EEG pattern is rarely seen in the extratemporal lobe epilepsies.

Frequently because much of the frontal lobe is underrepresented by scalp electrodes, ictal scalp EEG recordings in frontal lobe epilepsy may be nonlocalized and are often nonlateralized. Anterior frontal and dorsolateral frontal lobe seizure onset may be associated with focal repetitive IEDs. Focal electrographic seizures associated with rhythmic ictal fast activity greater than 13 Hz may be localizing and portend a more favorable outcome after resective surgery. Note the focal ictal onset manifest by beta frequencies in the patient above with lesional frontal lobe epilepsy (evident at FP1). High frequency oscillations in the gamma range (30–80 Hz) or even higher bandwidths involving ripples (80–250 Hz) and fast ripples (250–500 Hz) may be localizing.

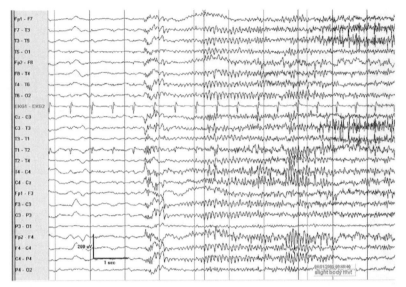

FIGURE 5.14. Nonlocalized ictal EEG in frontal lobe epilepsy. Notice the brief right frontal-centrally predominant burst of repetitive spikes during seconds 7 and 8.

Frontal lobe epilepsy often has very brief, bizarre, bimanual-bipedal automatisms with nocturnal predominance and be prone to acute repetitive seizures and status epilepticus. It is the second most common location in large epilepsy surgery series. Ictal scalp EEG is often of limited utility. In orbitofrontal and mesial frontal onset, seizures may have no representation at all or be obscured by an overriding muscle artifact to make scalp EEG "invisible" during the seizure. Interictal IEDs are notably absent in 30% of patients with frontal lobe epilepsy. Orbitofrontal and mesial frontal may not manifest interictal or ictal discharges due to their distance from recording scalp electrodes. Application of additional and midline electrodes may provide extra information in cases of frontal lobe seizures though precise localization commonly necessitate the use of intracranial EEG.

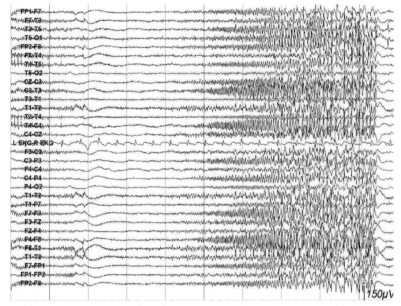

FIGURE 5.15. Scalp ictal EEG demonstrating an initial diffuse electrodecremental response in a patient with a supplementary motor seizure.

Supplementary motor seizures are seizures that begin in the mesial frontal lobe and often are associated with brief and bizarre semiologies that mimic psychogenic nonepileptic seizures (PNES) (pseudo-pseudoseizures). The clinical semiology is often nonlateralized though seizures may also manifest a "fencer's" posture that can provide more lateralizing with the side of tonic extension reflecting the side of involvement opposite to the hemisphere of seizure onset. Semiology and even brain MRI (when it demonstrates a discrete structural lesion) may provide a greater value for diagnostic localization than scalp ictal EEG (Figures 5.14 and 5.15). Seizures in mesial frontal lobe epilepsy are typically nonlocalized and are often nonlateralized with a significant minority that do not have detectable ictal EEG at all that are identifiable with scalp ictal EEG recording.

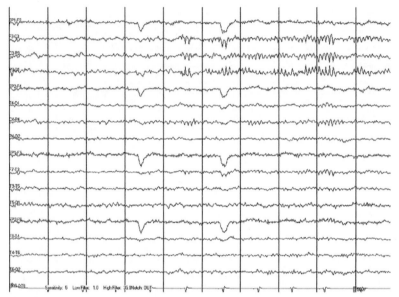

FIGURE 5.16. The tracing shows high-frequency, mu-like arcuate waveforms focally over the left parietal C3-P3 derivations at 10 Hz in the region of a brain tumor.

Parietal lobe seizures are often clinically silent. Somatosensory involvement may yield a perception of tingling, formication, pain, heat, movement, or dysmorphopsia, typically of the distal limb or face. As in frontal lobe epilepsy, only a small number of those with parietal ictal onset are focal. Minimal scalp EEG ictal changes may occur, and nonlateralized ictal onsets or even false lateralization occurring with parietal lobe epilepsy are not uncommon. Following seizure onset, propagation may occur to the supplementary motor area or temporal area and result in false electrographic lateralization or even localization due to a propagated EEG pattern that occurs after seizure onset. The patient above noted paroxysmal right arm and leg tingling during the recording.

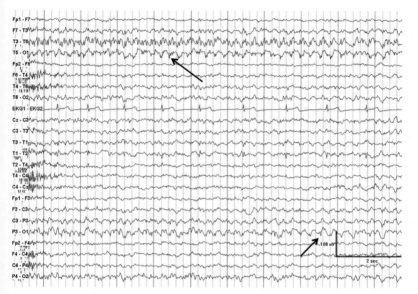

FIGURE 5.17. Left occipital seizure with right flashing lights, a feeling of doom, and late right eye deviation. Note the rhythmic 4 to 5 Hz theta with intermixed low amplitude surface negative spikes maximal at O1 (arrows).

Occipital lobe seizures are commonly manifest as visual dysfunction with phosphenes, unformed visual hallucinations, and less frequently blindness or hemianopsia that may occur. There may also be illusions where objects appear larger (macropsia), smaller (micropsia), distorted (metamorphopsia), or persistent after the visual stimulus (pallinopsia). High-frequency discharges at the temporoparieto-occipital junction can induce contralateral horizontal nystagmus and versive eye and head deviation. The EEG may show build-up of rapid alpha-beta activity focally over the temporoparieto-occipital junction or more posteriorly (see above), often with spread anteriorly within the posterior quadrant of the brain to the temporal structures as the seizure evolves from a focal seizure to a convulsion.

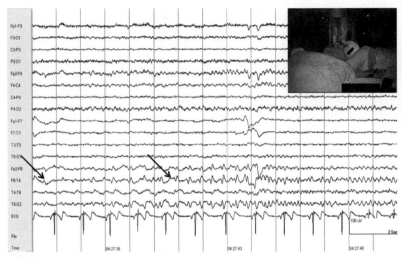

FIGURE 5.18. A subclinical seizure (arrows) in a patient with seizures without awareness captured during outpatient computer-assisted ambulatory EEG.

Subclinical seizures are an artifact of testing with the degree of "subclinical" occurrence reflecting the sophistication of behavioral test. Some seizures may occur without awareness or be so subtle that clinical signs are not observed. Temporal lobe seizures without awareness may mimic subclinical seizures unless responsiveness is adequately assessed during the event. When testing is performed during subclinical seizures, no evidence of interruption in behavior or consciousness is evident. In the patient above the clinical history suggested seizures without awareness in a patient with clinical focal seizures. An ambulatory EEG was performed to evaluate driving eligibility in a patient with seizures without awareness who self-reported seizure-freedom.

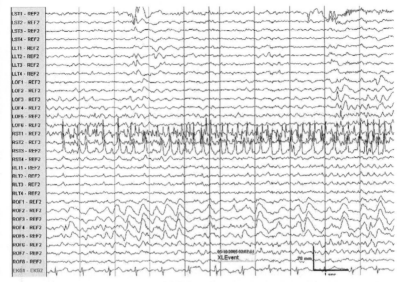

FIGURE 5.19. Right "focal" temporal seizure on intracranial EEG confined to the right subtemporal (RST) 1 to 3 electrodes following a poorly localized scalp ictal EEG. L(R) ST = left (right) subtemporal; L(R)LT = left (right) lateral temporal; L(R)OF = left (right) orbitofrontal.

Intracranial EEG may be necessary when localization is ill-defined on scalp EEG during the presurgical evaluation of drug-resistant epilepsy. Focal seizures may originate from one to two electrodes at seizure onset. Those seizures with a "focal" origin on the intracranial EEG imply a restricted generator adjacent to the recording electrode. In Figure 5.19, RST1 demonstrated an abrupt onset of rhythmic ictal frequencies greater than 13 Hz prior to RST1-3 repetitive spiking that remained a well-localized unilateral discharge for 20 sec prior to contralateral involvement of the left hemisphere. The "focal" onset, location, and prolonged unilateral involvement prior to propagation are favorable features for localizing seizures onset and predicting a favorable response to resective surgery. Following right temporal lobectomy, the patient has been seizure free.

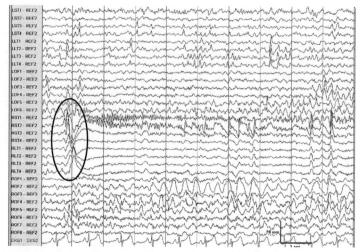

FIGURE 5.20. Right "regional" temporal onset (oval) in a patient suspected to have right frontal lobe epilepsy with seizure onset in the right subtemporal (RST) and right lateral temporal (RLT) subdural strip electrodes. L(R)ST = left (right) subtemporal; L(R)LT = left (right) lateral temporal; L(R)OF = left (right) orbitofrontal.

Regional onsets in patients with TLE identified by intracranial electrodes demonstrate more widespread areas of ictal onset. Lateralization and regionalization of the ictal activity are then complementary to the remaining parameters of the presurgical evaluation to demonstrate concordance for the purposes of epilepsy surgery. In the above EEG, note the large sharply contoured slow wave and regional attenuation in the right subtemporal (RST) and right lateral temporal (RLT) strips and rhythmic ictal fast activity in RST 1 and 2 at seizure onset.

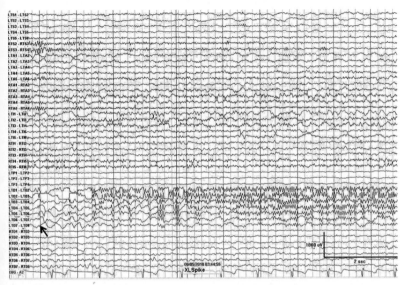

FIGURE 5.21. Focal seizure with onset in the left temporal depth electrode. Note the progressive spread from the initial onset of a single sentinel spike (arrow) to the gradual propagation of the rhythmic ictal fast activity.

Depth electrodes may be used to differentiate buried cortex that is inaccessible to subdural strips or grids of electrodes. Depths are commonly used for lateralization and delineation of patients suspected to have mesial TLE. Depth electrodes are commonly used with subdural strip or grid recordings (Figure 5.21). The use of depth electrodes in neocortical epilepsy has generated interest in the use of stereo-electroencephalography where multiple intracortical electrodes are used to define the dimensions of both the surface and the depth of the epileptogenic zone.

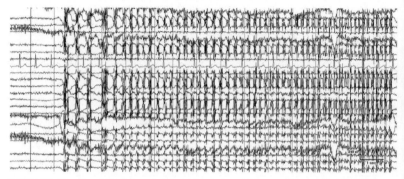

FIGURE 5.22. "Ictal" EEG in a patient with psychogenic nonepileptic seizure (PNES). Note the pseudo-"evolution" of rhythmic myogenic artifact that occurred from repetitive jaw movement to mimic an epileptic seizure on EEG. The patient was looking at the video-EEG monitor while this was produced.

As expected, the EEG during a psychogenic nonepileptic seizure (PNES) is normal. The importance of defining seizures as epileptic or nonepileptic is reflected in the significant number of patients with nonepileptic events that mimic epilepsy. PNES account for 20% to 30% of the admissions to hospital-based epilepsy monitoring units and are about as prevalent as multiple sclerosis.

Overinterpretation of EEG patterns that are normal is a common substrate for misdiagnosis. An artifact may be the culprit leading to a false diagnosis of epilepsy. In the example above, compare the similarity of the pattern in Figure 5.22 with "pseudoevolution" to Figure 5.5 that occurs with a generalized epileptic seizure.

ADDITIONAL RESOURCES

Benbadis SR. The EEG of nonepileptic seizures. *J Clin Neurophysiol*. 2006;23:340-352.

Blume WT, Holloway GM, Wiebe S. Temporal epileptogenesis: localizing value of scalp and subdural interictal and ictal EEG data. *Epilepsia*. 2000;42:508-514.

Farrell K, Tatum WO. Encephalopathic generalized epilepsy and Lennox-Gastaut syndrome. In: Wyllie E, ed. *The Treatment of Epilepsy; Practice and Principals*. 4th ed. Baltimore, MD: Lippincott Williams & Williams; 2006:429-440.

Foldvary N, Klem G, Hammel J, Bingaman W, Najm I, Lüders H. The localizing value of ictal EEG in focal epilepsy. *Neurology*. 2001;57:2022-2028.

Olivier D, Blauwblomme T, Job AS, et al. Imaging the seizure-onset zone with stereo-electroencephalography. *Brain*. 2011;134(10):2898-2911.

Pacia SV, Ebersole JS. Intracranial EEG substrates of scalp ictal patterns from temporal lobe foci. *Epilepsia*. 1997;38:642-654.

So, EL. Value and limitations of seizure semiology in localizing seizure onset. *J Clin Neurophysiol*. 2006;23:353-357.

Tatum WO IV. Long-term EEG monitoring: a clinical approach to electrophysiology. *J Clin Neurophysiol*. 2001;18(5):442-455.

Tatum WO, Ho S, Benbadis SR. Polyspike ictal onset absence seizures. *J Clin Neurophysiol*. 2010;27(2):93-99.

Verma A, Radtke R. EEG of partial seizures. *J Clin Neurophysiol*. 2006;23:333-339.

Westmoreland BF. The EEG findings in extratemporal seizures. *Epilepsia*. 1998; 39(suppl 4):S1-S8.

Worrell GA, Parish L, Cranstoun SD, Ionas R, Baltuch G, Litt B. High-frequency oscillations and seizure generation in neocortical epilepsy. *Brain*. 2004;127:1496-1506.

6

The EEG in Status Epilepticus

Frank W. Drislane,
William O. Tatum, IV, and
Peter W. Kaplan

Status epilepticus (SE) is a prolonged seizure or a series of seizures without recovery between them. There are many forms of SE, with different clinical and electrographic (EEG) manifestations. Deciding which type of SE a patient has is important in directing proper management and in predicting the outcome. EEG is often a crucial part of that evaluation.

Both convulsive and nonconvulsive forms of SE occur. Generalized convulsive status epilepticus (GCSE) is the best described type of SE and has the greatest morbidity, mortality, and clinical urgency for treatment. GCSE must be diagnosed and treated promptly, in part for concern that it may become refractory to treatment and have grave consequences. On the other hand, there is little evidence that most nonconvulsive status epilepticus (NCSE) causes lasting neurologic harm. In the case of NCSE, the treatment imperative is, therefore, less, but not negligible. NCSE has been referred to as "underdiagnosed and over-treated." Continuous EEG recording can help elucidate the temporal pattern of recurrent seizures when subtle or no clinical signs are evident.

GENERALIZED CONVULSIVE STATUS EPILEPTICUS

Clinical and EEG manifestations of generalized convulsions and GCSE are usually symmetric from the onset, although some may exhibit focal or lateralizing features (Figure 6.1). On the EEG, the seizure typically begins with bilaterally symmetric epileptiform discharges. The initial sudden interruption in behavior is often accompanied by widespread voltage attenuation or desynchronization, with faster frequencies between 20 and 40 Hz introduced into the background and producing an "electrodecremental" appearance of the ictal EEG. This is often the time when myogenic artifact obscures the EEG recording of the tonic and clonic phases of a convulsion, although sometimes, epileptiform discharges may be evident at the vertex. The superimposed EMG activity itself may exhibit a characteristic rhythmic appearance in synchrony with the clinical features of repetitive clonic jerks.

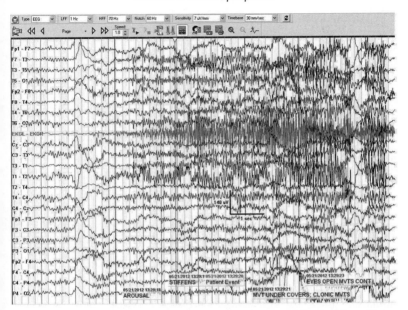

FIGURE 6.1. GCSE begins with a lower voltage faster frequency pattern, followed by prominent muscle artifact (on the right side of figure). © WO Tatum, 2013.

Following an individual seizure, repetitive epileptiform discharges (EDs) may decrease from several per second to a frequency less than 1 Hz. The discharges might not disappear entirely, giving way to generalized periodic discharges (GPDs) or lateralized periodic discharges (LPDs), usually on a suppressed background, for at least several minutes before the gradual return of a normal background—or prior to another convulsion if GCSE has not been terminated.

When GCSE is prolonged, the EEG becomes more discontinuous, and clinical manifestations may become minimal. When the visible motor manifestations of SE cease, this may be termed "subtle" GCSE. At this point, clinical signs are minimal and may include low amplitude eyelid or facial twitching, intermittent myoclonic jerks, repetitive or sustained nystagmus, or even the absence of all clinical movement. Persistence of regular and rhythmic GPDs that are 3 Hz or greater suggests that nonconvulsive seizures are still ongoing and that the SE has become refractory despite the lack of clinical signs. At this stage, patients are typically comatose.

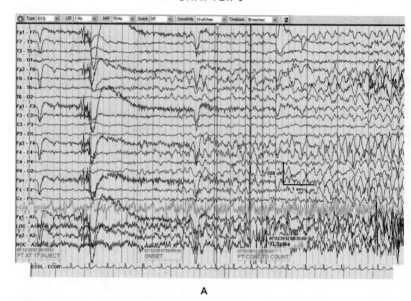

A

FIGURE 6.2. (A) Seizures begin with rhythmic slowing in right-sided channels, spreading bilaterally. (B) Discrete seizures merge and become continuous, primarily over the right hemisphere. (C) Seizures are continuous, still primarily over the right hemisphere. (D) Seizure activity is interrupted by episodes of a suppressed background. (E) The background becomes more suppressed, and discharges recur with a longer periodicity. © WO Tatum, 2013.

Some have proposed that there is a characteristic sequence of EEG changes during GCSE—based on EEG recordings taken from animals and humans at various stages of (usually generalized convulsive) SE. This sequence of EEG changes (Figure 6.2) includes: (A) Discrete seizures that are repetitive and separated electrographically by background slowing and attenuation in between recurrent seizures. (B) Seizures that merge gradually, with some fluctuation in voltage and frequency. (C) Continuous seizure activity, but sometimes with asymmetric ictal discharges, reflecting the focal or lateralized onset of many seizures. (D) Ongoing seizure activity interrupted by brief periods of a suppressed background, often for just a second or so. (E) In late SE, the background becomes suppressed, with GPDs or infrequent bursts of polyspikes (see Figures 6.2E and 6.3). "Subtle" SE often corresponds to EEG stages D and E.

(Continued)

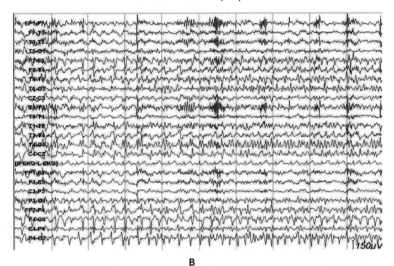

B

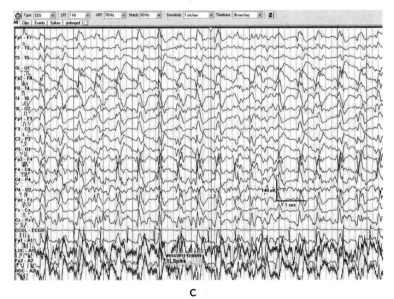

C

FIGURE 6.2. (*Continued*)

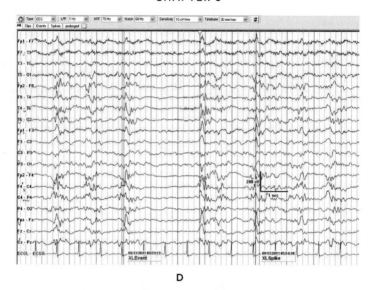

D

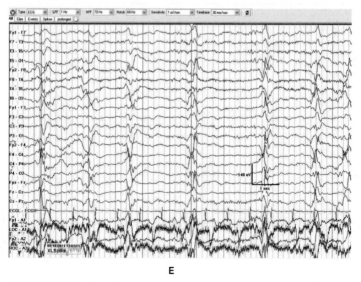

E

FIGURE 6.2. (*Continued*)

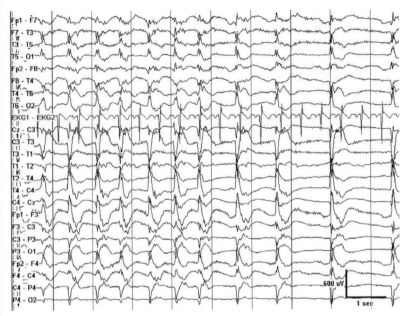

FIGURE 6.3. Following a seizure, there are generalized periodic discharges (GPDs), gradually decreasing in frequency.

While the later phases of this EEG sequence are thought to reflect the uncoupling of the electrical and mechanical activity after prolonged SE, not all clinical neurophysiologists have found such a predictable or homogeneous sequence of EEG patterns in many patients. Still, these patterns are often useful in determining the approximate phase of SE a patient is in, and whether the SE is prolonged enough (electrographically, when not evident clinically) that treatment for refractory SE should be considered.

FOCAL MOTOR STATUS EPILEPTICUS

There are many causes of focal motor status epilepticus (FMSE). Stroke (ischemic or hemorrhagic) is by far the most common cause. SE occurs in about 1% of all acute strokes, although isolated seizures are substantially more common. Central nervous system infection (e.g., meningoencephalitis) is another common cause. Herpes simplex encephalitis may be manifested clinically as FMSE. Other etiologies of FMSE include vasculitis, mass lesions, trauma, multiple sclerosis, and, rarely, mitochondrial or degenerative disorders. Occasionally, benign idiopathic focal epilepsies, such as benign childhood epilepsy with centrotemporal spikes (Rolandic epilepsy) can lead to FMSE. Seizures in these benign syndromes are typically infrequent, often treated easily, and seldom lead to SE.

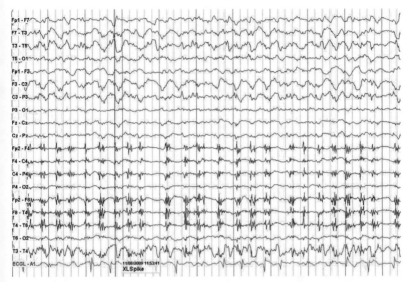

FIGURE 6.4. Focal motor status epilepticus with intact consciousness, with semi-rhythmic slowing and sharp features over the left hemisphere, and EMG artifact from facial twitching on the right. © WO Tatum, 2013.

In focal motor SE, the features found on ictal EEG are quite variable (Figure 6.4). Epileptiform activity may consist of discrete, frequently recurrent focal motor seizures that are localized or lateralized to one hemisphere or have an asymmetric bihemispheric involvement when consciousness is impaired. There may be clinical recovery between seizures, or there may be continuous electrographic seizure activity. Following individual focal seizures, or between electrographic focal seizures on EEG, there may be continued slowing or LPDs. In terms of diagnosis and clinical outcome, there does not appear to be a large difference between the discrete and continuous forms of FMSE.

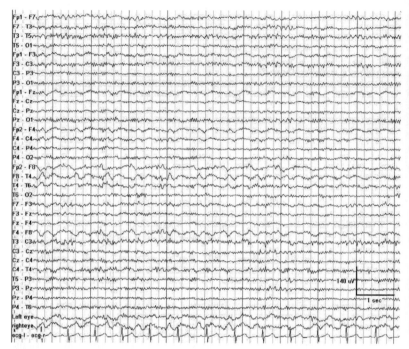

FIGURE 6.5. Epilepsia partialis continua (EPC) in a 41 year old patient with a sense of 'tingling' and twitching on the left side of the mouth. Note primarily the rhythmic delta slowing, phase reversing at F8.

Clinically, FMSE may be manifested as prolonged regular jerking of an isolated area of the body such as the face, hand, or foot. This is referred to as *epilepsia partialis continua* (EPC) (Figure 6.5). EPC can last days or weeks. Almost always, there is a responsible focal lesion, but there is not always an identifiable focal rhythmic ED on the surface EEG. Although repetitive EDs or rhythmic theta or delta slowing are also common patterns with EPC, some epileptic foci are generated in deeper "buried" cortex; have limited surface area involved (i.e., less than 10 cm^2); or have a dipolar source that is not oriented "favorably" for detection by surface electrodes, so there is often minimal or no change detected on surface EEG despite ongoing focal seizures.

(Continued)

LPDs (see also Chapter 7) are repetitive spike or sharp and slow wave complexes. They usually last 100 to 400 msec and typically recur at 0.5 to 2 Hz but sometimes have longer intervals. They are usually distributed broadly over most of one hemisphere, with an attenuated EEG background between discharges. Most epileptologists do not consider LPDs to be clinical seizures or SE per se, but rather an epiphenomenon that is usually associated with acute, serious neurologic illness affecting the gray matter. In about 90% of cases there is a structural lesion. Stroke is the most common cause, although tumor, and occasionally, CNS infections, and severe metabolic disturbances may result in LPDs. Some epilepsy may also exhibit LPDs as an interictal or ictal phenomenon. In many cases, LPDs may be considered "the terminal phase of status epilepticus."

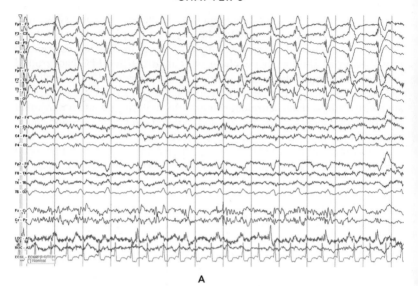

A

FIGURE 6.6. The EEG of a 41-year-old man with a metastatic tumor shows periodic lateralized discharges over the left hemisphere (A). Discharges become more complex, with frequent after-going low-voltage fast activity (B). The "LPDs+" are followed by brief bursts of electrographic seizure activity at about 3 Hz (C). © F Drislane, 2012; courtesy of the author.

While most LPDs are manifested on the EEGs as EDs recurring every 1 to 2 seconds, some intervals may be 10 seconds or longer. The more rapid discharges of 3 Hz or faster are a definite EEG correlate of seizures, but most electroencephalographers consider that there is a significant risk of ongoing seizures when the frequency of LPDs exceeds 1.5 to 2.0 Hz. "LPDs+" is a term describing LPDs that are associated with a low voltage rhythmic epileptiform discharge or other rhythmic pattern occurring between the high voltage periodic discharges. LPDs+ are more likely to be associated with epileptic seizures than are "LPDs proper" (Figure 6.6).

(Continued)

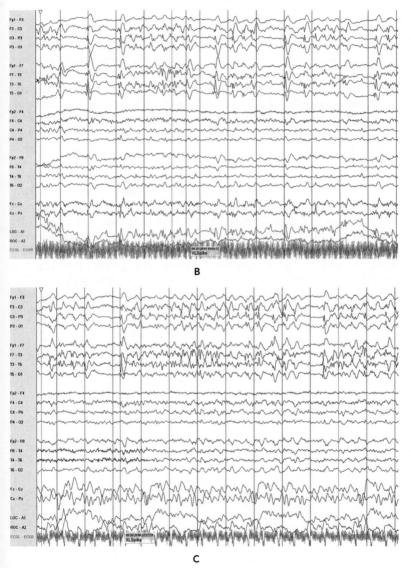

B

C

FIGURE 6.6. (Continued)

MYOCLONIC STATUS EPILEPTICUS

Myoclonic status epilepticus (MSE) has many etiologies and occurs in many different epilepsy syndromes. Although the clinical appearance of recurrent lightening-like jerks may be similar, there are many different MSE syndromes. Many cases of MSE occur in patients with one of the Genetic (idiopathic) Generalized Epilepsies (GGEs), or primary epilepsy syndromes. In this case, interictal myoclonus is common, typically consisting of a sudden quick muscular jerk involving primarily the upper body and often occurring in repetitive clusters. Myoclonus may involve eyelid myoclonia alone (e.g., in Jeavon's syndrome). Common childhood GGEs include juvenile absence epilepsy and juvenile myoclonic epilepsy. The frequency of MSE is syndrome-dependent. MSE may occur following sleep deprivation, exposure to toxins (e.g., alcohol), when concentrations of anti-seizure drugs (ASDs) are low, (e.g., noncompliance), or if ASDs inappropriate for particular GGEs are used (e.g., carbamazepine or phenytoin). In MSE, consciousness may be preserved, even when myoclonic jerks are frequent. The EEG demonstrates EDs of 3 Hz or greater. Typically, "fast" (greater than 3 Hz, but less than 6 Hz) generalized, symmetric, bifrontally-predominant polyspike-and-waves and generalized spike-and-waves accompany the myoclonic jerks. With protracted duration or during drowsiness, lateralizing features on the EEG may be accentuated.

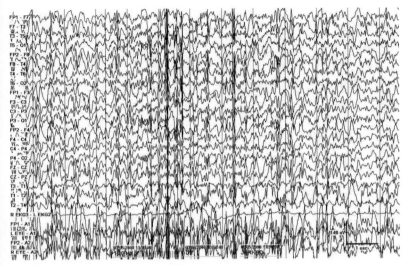

FIGURE 6.7. EEG during myoclonic status epilepticus in Lafora body disease. There are frequent spike discharges with a generalized distribution, but they are often difficult to distinguish from muscle or movement artifact. © WO Tatum, 2013.

"Secondary" MSE is often the manifestation of serious, widespread underlying brain dysfunction, including the 'progressive myoclonus epilepsies," some of which are caused by storage diseases such as Lafora disease (Figure 6.7). These syndromes also include severe infant and pediatric conditions such as Lennox-Gastaut syndrome, in which other seizures such as "myoclonic astatic" seizures occur. MSE is more common in these epilepsy syndromes than in the GGEs.

The EEG helps to distinguish the different types of MSE, providing information on the underlying brain function and often, a guide to optimal treatment. In the GGE syndromes, the EEG during myoclonic seizures typically demonstrates rapid (~4 Hz) generalized, frontally predominant polyspikes on a normal background, although in MSE, the background activity may become slow due to the frequent seizures or from the effect of medication. Sometimes, the spikes occur just before the clinical myoclonic jerk (Figure 6.7). In this case, the interictal EEG may show a normal background, with frequent spikes and polyspikes. In the "secondary" epilepsy syndromes, the spike and wave discharges are often "slow" (i.e., 2–2.5 Hz). Finally, in "symptomatic" types of MSE, there is usually an underlying encephalopathy reflected by diffuse slowing of all background activity. For example, in the MSE that follows anoxia, the EEG background is usually slow and of very low voltage, auguring very poorly for prognosis. In this case, the underlying pathophysiologic mechanism of MSE may well differ significantly from that in the various epilepsy syndromes described earlier.

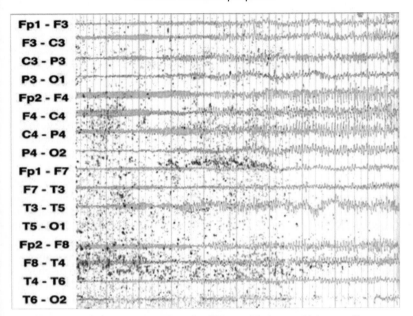

FIGURE 6.8. EEG during a tonic seizure in a 50-year-old woman with Lennox-Gastaut syndrome, with preserved consciousness during the seizures, recurring several times each minute. This image of a paper EEG shows scattering of ink from the "violent" higher frequency activity of the ink pens. This episode of tonic SE worsened with benzodiazepines but improved with phenytoin. Courtesy, P Kaplan, MD.

Tonic status epilepticus (TSE) is rare in adults. It consists of maintenance of a tonic posture, particularly of axial musculature, rather than of recurrent convulsions. The EEG often shows widespread fast activity or very rapid spikes. Sometimes, periods of background suppression or attenuation (Figure 6.8) may be evident.

NONCONVULSIVE STATUS EPILEPTICUS

NCSE has protean manifestations and many etiologies. Many cases of NCSE are characterized by impairment of alertness, attention, cognition, or behavior relative to baseline function. Observable signs may be subtle, with minimal automatisms or myoclonus as the only motor manifestation. NCSE may include primarily sensory symptoms, language deficits such as aphasia, psychiatric manifestations, and even autonomic features (e.g., in the Panayiotopoulos syndrome). There are many conditions other than epilepsy that can cause altered alertness or behavior, and NCSE can be very difficult to recognize; the EEG is crucial for diagnosis.

In early reports, NCSE was oversimplified into "absence" SE [if NCSE was associated with GSW on the EEG], and "complex partial" SE [if there were focal EDs on the EEG or a clear focal onset was noted clinically]. Currently, NCSE may be divided into SE with a focal onset and NCSE with generalized discharges and nonfocal clinical features. The latter, however, should be divided further into generalized NCSE occurring in patients with GGE (including absence SE) and the remainder with generalized discharges that are presumably associated with focal origins and are secondarily generalized.

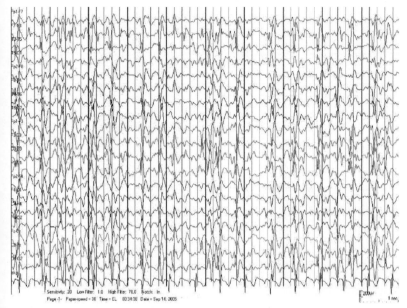

FIGURE 6.9. Electrical status epilepticus in sleep (ESES) in a 9-year-old boy with Landau–Kleffner syndrome. The EEG shows generalized discharges that are not always rhythmic.

NCSE among neonates and infants has remarkably different clinical manifestations and EEG patterns from those in children and adults. Some occur in the "epileptic encephalopathies" in which infants or young children have severe encephalopathies associated with very frequent interictal EDs on EEG, but in which the EEG pattern and the clinical seizures do not always correlate well. One example is electrical status epilepticus in sleep (ESES) (Figure 6.9) in which clinical seizures may be absent from the epilepsy syndrome. ESES denotes a marked activation of EDs, occupying the majority of the EEG and suggesting SE, during N3 sleep. The waking EEG usually shows focal or occasionally generalized interictal EDs with the spike component usually more prominent than the slow wave.

FOCAL NONCONVULSIVE STATUS EPILEPTICUS

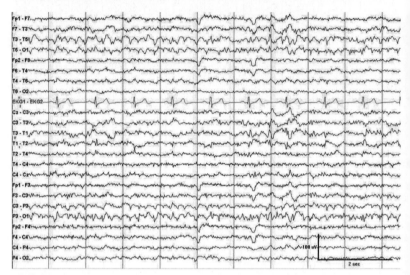

FIGURE 6.10. A patient with ongoing left occipital SE manifested by persistent visual hallucinations of colored spheres in the right visual field without impairment of consciousness. © WO Tatum, 2013.

Focal NCSE has a variety of clinical features that may include sensory, visual, auditory, or olfactory symptoms that may appear to represent nonepileptic hallucinations (Figure 6.10). Manifestations may also be autonomic, psychic, or cognitive, with impairment of attention, language, mood, or behavior.

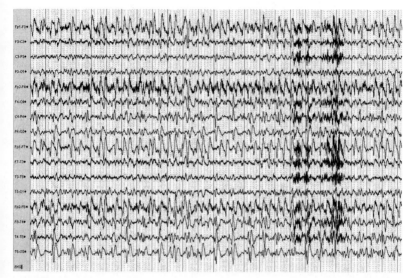

FIGURE 6.11. Focal SE with impaired consciousness (complex partial SE) in a 21-year-old patient following an episode of encephalitis. The primary symptom was confusion. Epileptiform activity is noted over the right hemisphere. © WO Tatum, 2013.

The persistence or recurrence of focal seizures with dyscognitive features is probably the most common form of NCSE in adults; most of these are considered complex partial status epilepticus (CPSE). Focal SE usually begins with a focal-onset seizure and progresses to include an alteration in consciousness (i.e., responsiveness). Seizures may be continuous or may wax and wane, with fluctuating clinical manifestations. The EEG in focal SE with impaired consciousness (complex partial SE) develops over time, with repetitive focal-onset seizures in which epileptiform discharges may merge gradually to produce continuous focal seizure activity (Figure 6.11). During a seizure, the discharges tend to increase in voltage and later slow in frequency. Many seizures have subsequent spread to involve a greater area of the cortex, and some spread to generalized EDs or potentially even to clinical convulsions. Between discrete seizures there may be repetitive or periodic focal discharges and focal slowing before the next seizure begins.

GENERALIZED NONCONVULSIVE STATUS EPILEPTICUS

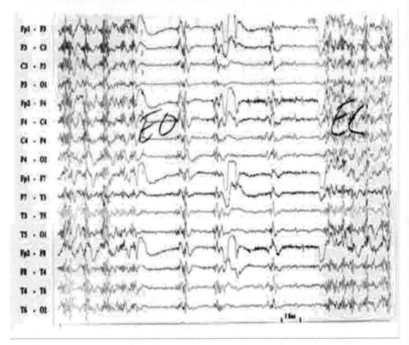

FIGURE 6.12. Fixation-off absence SE in a 25-year-old woman with earlier absence epilepsy beginning at age 8. In adulthood, she had episodes of eye blinking, staring, and slurred, interrupted speech. EO=eyes open and EC=eyes closed. Courtesy, P Kaplan, MD.

SE is relatively infrequent in the GGEs, but there are several GGE syndromes that can lead to SE (Figure 6.12). They may present as ongoing seizures lasting more than 5 minutes and often tend to continue beyond 30 minutes in duration, the traditional definition of SE. SE is thought to occur when the self-sustaining processes causing seizures prevail over the self-terminating mechanisms.

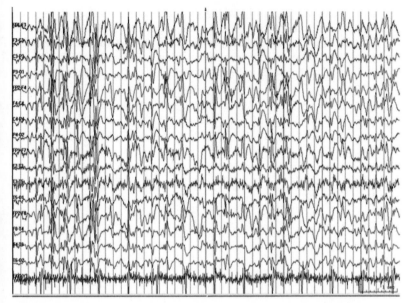

FIGURE 6.13. A 40-year-old woman with Jeavon's syndrome, including eye blinking. The patient had the onset of absence seizures as a child, with myoclonic and generalized convulsive seizures in adolescence and frequent hospitalizations throughout adulthood. At the time, she was evaluated for confusion with eyelid myoclonia. The EEG shows prolonged bursts of nearly continuous generalized spikes and polyspikes. Courtesy, P Kaplan, MD.

The clinical expression of SE in the GGEs includes absence SE; tonic-clonic (or convulsive) SE; clonic SE; tonic SE (a debatable entity); and myoclonic forms of SE. Absence SE is the classic and most common form of GGE, followed by tonic-clonic SE, and then MSE (as in cases of juvenile myoclonic epilepsy). In all types of GGE, SE usually arises from insufficient or inappropriate ASDs or from behavioral triggers that lower the seizure threshold. Absence SE or MSE may terminate in a generalized convulsion. Absence SE may last from hours to over a week. MSE usually lasts less than a day, waxing and waning over the course. With both absence SE and MSE, the patient may be awake and appear alert, but detailed testing may demonstrate variable impairment of abstract thinking, personal awareness, and other higher cortical function. Some absence SE includes frequent eyelid myoclonias, with or without GSWs (e.g., Jeavon's syndrome) (Figure 6.13).

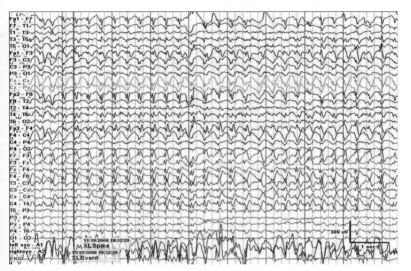

FIGURE 6.14. Typical absence SE in a 38-year-old with a history of juvenile myoclonic epilepsy. Discharges are very regular. © WO Tatum, 2013.

"True" or "typical" absence SE occurs in patients with absence epilepsy. Of all types of NCSE, this is a relatively small minority, but easily recognizable. Typical clinical manifestations include confusion, with occasional minimal motor abnormalities such as blinking or myoclonus, or brief, minimal automatisms. On EEG, very regular and stereotyped generalized, bifrontally predominant 3 Hz spike-and-slow-waves occur in prolonged runs. The EDs of absence SE may occur at a frequency of up to 4 Hz, especially at the onset (Figure 6.14). Rhythmic repetitive generalized EDs on the EEG also occur in other GGEs and are not specific for an individual GGE syndrome.

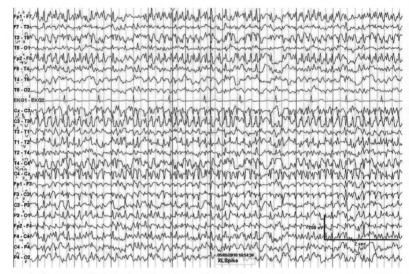

FIGURE 6.15. Rhythmic 4 to 6 Hz spike and slow wave activity of *de novo* absence SE in a 78-year-old with no clinical signs except impaired responsiveness. © WO Tatum, 2013.

Relatively frequent episodes of NCSE have been reported in older patients without epilepsy ("*de novo* absence SE of late onset"), some in association with withdrawal of benzodiazepines. Some such patients may have had some features of a GGE earlier in life but have remained undiagnosed. In *de novo* absence SE, EEG discharges are often less rhythmic and regular than those in patients with typical absence SE (Figure 6.15), but they are usually generalized and rapid. *De novo* absence SE often responds quickly to benzodiazepine treatment, even in low doses.

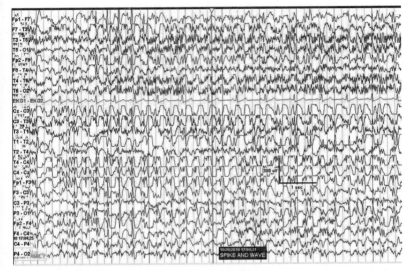

FIGURE 6.16. Atypical absence SE with a slower (2.5 Hz) spike and wave pattern and intermixed fast activity. © WO Tatum, 2013.

Atypical absence SE (AASE) is infrequent and occurs primarily in children with frequent seizures of mixed types. AASE may be manifested as a change in the baseline mental status or level of alertness. An underlying severe encephalopathy with frequent seizures, such as Lennox Gastaut syndrome (LGS), is common. These conditions often include multiple seizure types (including tonic and myoclonic seizures), and severe developmental delay and neurocognitive impairment. In most patients, the baseline EEG shows a widespread slow background, with frequent, generalized or multifocal spike discharges. Ictally, there is often a characteristic "slow spike and wave" (SSW) repetitive discharge at 1 to 2.5 Hz. In early childhood, the SSW may occur in prolonged runs and suggest AASE, but without clear clinical signs of seizures and rather, just a subtle decline in mental status. The SSW on EEG is key to the diagnosis of LGS, but this pattern may be lost in adults. AASE has less rhythmicity and symmetry than is seen in typical ASE (Figure 6.16).

ELECTROGRAPHIC STATUS EPILPETICUS

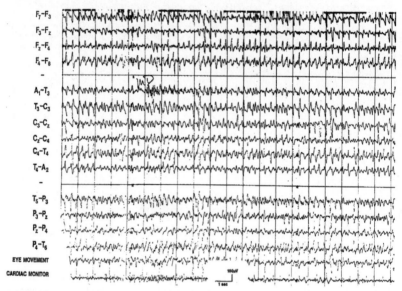

FIGURE 6.17. Continuous 3-Hz generalized epileptiform discharges in an 83-year-old woman found to be stuporous after admission to the hospital, but without a clear cause. © F Drislane, 2009; courtesy of the author.

Most NCSE in hospital settings is secondarily generalized from a focal onset, often due to an underlying structural lesion (Figure 6.17). Nevertheless, the clinical manifestation can be simply an impairment of alertness or responsiveness. The generalized EDs on EEG may not indicate a clear focal seizure origin even when there is a focal lesion; there may be a deeper focus and rapid generalization. Detection of this type of SE is one of the primary goals of continuous EEG monitoring in the intensive care unit (ICU), where nonconvulsive seizures and NCSE are captured frequently on EEG without apparent clinical signs.

The EEG in Status Epilepticus

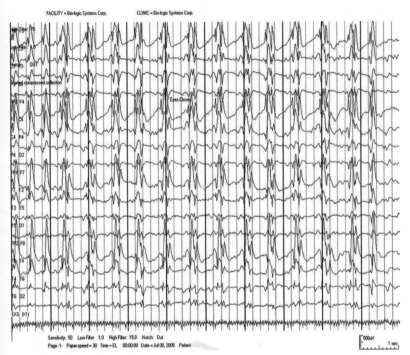

FIGURE 6.18. SE due to anoxia in a 50-year-old following cardiac arrest and hypothermia. The suppressed background between discharges augurs for an unfavorable prognosis. Courtesy, P Kaplan, MD.

This ongoing electrographic seizure activity, often following the apparent termination of prior generalized convulsions or GCSE (usually with minimal or no motor convulsive activity) may be termed "electrographic status epilepticus" (ESE). It typically occurs in the setting of severe medical illness such as sepsis, anoxia or severe metabolic derangements and is the most common type of NCSE in special care units, including the ICU (Figures 6.18 and 6.19). It has been referred to as "status epilepticus in coma," but not all such patients are comatose; most have severe medical and neurologic illnesses. ESE is often found in patients with severely abnormal mental status but in whom the SE was unsuspected before the EEG.

CHALLENGING DIAGNOSES

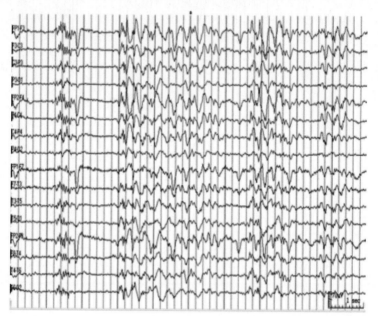

FIGURE 6.19. Case 1: A 41-year-old man with a generalized convulsion at age 34 was treated with valproate. The EEG was normal when the patient was asymptomatic. At a later clinic visit, he presented with chin tremor only. Courtesy, P Kaplan, MD.

Often, the most difficult problem in the management of SE is arriving at the correct diagnosis. Interpreting the EEG in the context of the clinical situation can be difficult. Some patterns (e.g., LPDs) have controversial clinical implications. There is also incomplete agreement, even among experienced electroencephalographers, concerning which EEGs are diagnostic of ongoing electrographic seizures and NCSE. The following figures illustrate potential pitfalls in interpreting the EEG, especially in critically ill patients (Figures 6.19 to 6.22) as discussed on page 187.

(Continued)

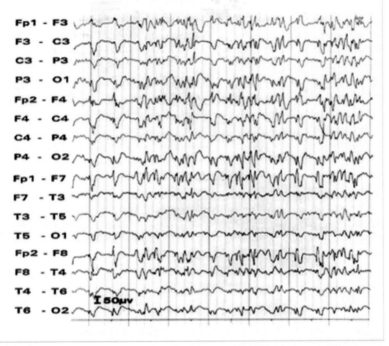

FIGURE 6.20. Case 2. A 54-year-old man with absence seizures as a child presents with prolonged confusional events in adulthood. Courtesy, P Kaplan, MD.

(Continued)

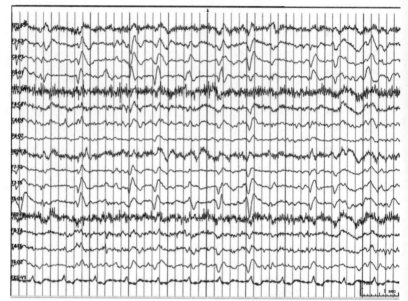

FIGURE 6.21. Case 3. An 82-year-old woman with hypothyroidism and a history of progressive dementia. The patient startled easily, but had no myoclonus, gait disturbance, or coordination problems. Courtesy, P Kaplan, MD.

(*Continued*)

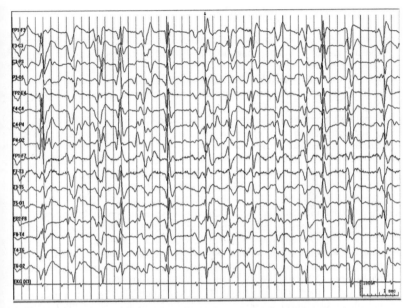

FIGURE 6.22. Case 4. A 75-year-old woman with episodes of confusion and unresponsiveness was found on the floor, unresponsive to any stimulation. Courtesy, P Kaplan, MD.

The first EEG (Figure 6.19) shows bursts of generalized spike- and polyspike-and-slow-wave discharges, supporting a diagnosis of NCSE. ASDs led to an improvement in the EEG and in the clinical condition. The second (Figure 6.20) has frequent repetitive EDs on the EEG, also suggesting NCSE. The spikes are regular, very brief, and have a generalized distribution typical for GGE. Figure 6.21 shows generalized periodic discharges—with left hemispheric predominance repeating at a frequency of less than 1 Hz. The frequency and lack of rhythmicity and evolution suggest that this is the sign of disordered brain function rather than a seizure, per se. This EEG was recorded from a patient with Creutzfeldt-Jakob disease who did not have NCSE. The final EEG (Figure 6.22) shows frequent, but not rhythmic, GPDs. This is not NCSE; the EEG features resulted from an overdose of baclofen.

CHAPTER 6

ADDITIONAL RESOURCES

Agathonikou A, Panayiotopoulos CP, Giannakodimos S, Koutroumanidis M. Typical absence status in adults: diagnostic and syndromic considerations. *Epilepsia.* 1998;39:1265-1276.

Claassen J, Mayer SA, Kowalski RG, Emerson RG, Hirsch LJ. Detection of electrographic seizures with continuous EEG monitoring in critically ill patients. *Neurology.* 2004;62:1743-1748.

Cockerell OC, Rothwell J, Thompson PD, Marsden CD, Shorvon SD. Clinical and physiological features of epilepsia partialis continua. Cases ascertained in the UK. *Brain.* 1996;119(Pt 2):393-407.

Devinsky O, Kelley K, Porter RJ, Theodore WH. Clinical and electroencephalographic features of simple partial seizures. *Neurology.* 1988;38:1347-1352.

Drislane FW, Blum AS, Schomer DL. Focal status epilepticus: clinical features and significance of different EEG patterns. *Epilepsia.* 1999;40:1254-1260.

Drislane FW, Herman ST, Kaplan RW. Convulsive status epilepticus. Chapter 28. In: Schomer DL, Lopes da Silva F, eds. *Niedermeyer's Electroencephalography.* 6th ed. Philadelphia, PA: Lippincott Williams & Wilkins; 2010:563-594.

Drislane FW, Kaplan PW, Herman ST. Nonconvulsive status epilepticus. Chapter 29. In: Schomer DL, Lopes da Silva F, eds. *Niedermeyer's Electroencephalography.* 6th ed. Philadelphia, PA: Lippincott Williams & Wilkins; 2010:595-643.

Husain AM, Horn GJ, Jacobson MP. Non-convulsive status epilepticus: usefulness of clinical features in selecting patients for urgent EEG. *J Neurol Neurosurg Psychiatry.* 2003;74:189-191.

Kaplan PW. Assessing the outcomes in patients with nonconvulsive status epilepticus: nonconvulsive status epilepticus is underdiagnosed, potentially overtreated, and confounded by comorbidity. *J Clin Neurophysiol.* 1999;16:341-352.

Manford M, Shorvon SD. Prolonged sensory or visceral symptoms: an underdiagnosed form of non-convulsive focal (simple partial) status epilepticus. *J Neurol Neurosurg Psychiatry.* 1992;55:714-716.

Ohtahara S, Ohtsuka Y. Myoclonic status epilepticus. Chapter 63. In: Engel J Jr, Pedley TA, eds. *Epilepsy: A Comprehensive Textbook.* 2nd ed. Philadelphia, PA: Lippincott-Raven Publishers; 2008:725-729.

Reiher J, Rivest J, Grand'Maison F, Leduc CP. Periodic lateralized epileptiform discharges with transitional rhythmic discharges: association with seizures. *Electroencephalogr Clin Neurophysiol.* 1991;78:12-17.

Panayiotopoulos CP. *A Clinical Guide to Epileptic Syndromes and Their Treatment.* 2nd ed. London; New York: Springer Healthcare; 2010.

Shorvon S, Walker M. Status epilepticus in idiopathic generalized epilepsy. *Epilepsia.* 2005;46:73-79.

Snodgrass SM, Tsuburaya K, Ajmone-Marsan C. Clinical significance of periodic lateralized epileptiform discharges: relationship with status epilepticus. *J Clin Neurophysiol.* 1989;6:159-172.

Thomas P, Beaumanoir A, Genton P, Dolisi C, Chatel M. "De novo" absence status of late onset: report of 11 cases. *Neurology.* 1992;42:104-110.

Tomson T, Svanborg E, Wedlund JE. Nonconvulsive status epilepticus: high incidence of complex partial status. *Epilepsia.* 1986;27:276-285.

Treiman DM, Walton NY, Kendrick C. A progressive sequence of electroencephalographic changes during generalized convulsive status epilepticus. *Epilepsy Res.* 1990;5:49-60.

7

ICU EEG

Nicolas Gaspard and Lawrence J. Hirsch

A s many as 10% to 20% of patients admitted to an ICU with altered mental status will have seizures, of which the majority are nonconvulsive and can only be detected with continuous EEG monitoring (CEEG). A similar proportion of patients will have periodic or stimulus-induced rhythmic discharges that are sometimes difficult to interpret as an ongoing seizure. The detection of these discharges is important as they may suggest a new focal abnormality of the brain that was not clinically evident, herald seizures at a later time during the CEEG, reflect nonconvulsive seizures (NCSz) or status epilepticus (SE) that becomes clearly delineated with prolonged recording time. The EEG may also suggest a specific diagnosis (e.g., lateralized period discharges (LPDs) according to the new American Clinical Neurophysiology terminology (see reference); formerly called periodic lateralized epileptiform discharges [PLEDs]" in herpes encephalitis, 1 Hz genealized periodic discharges (GPDs); formerly called generalized periodic epileptiform discharges (GPEDs) in Creutzfeldt-Jacob disease; extreme delta brushes in anti-NMDA encephalitis). There is significant variability and, therefore, controversy has been associated with the correct interpretation of the CEEG and the clinical implications of periodic and rhythmic patterns that occur in critically ill patients. The American Clinical Neurophysiology Society (ACNS) has developed a consensus terminology in an attempt to provide objective and well-defined terms for these patterns. In the following text we will use this terminology to describe the relevant features of CEEG, but will also include the older terms that correspond.

Information that is obtained from the EEG may also be useful in assessing and monitoring the degree of cerebral dysfunction, especially when the clinical examination is of limited utility (e.g., in comatose patients). The use of quantitative EEG and display of long-term trends is particularly helpful for condensing the data to allow a better appreciation of slowly evolving variations and long term trends that are difficult to notice at conventional "paper" speed. One example is the detection of delayed cerebral ischemia that develops late in the course after aneurysmal subarachnoid hemorrhage.

Nonepileptic motor manifestations that are misinterpreted as seizures may include clonus triggered by stretch of the deep tendons, tremor, posturing, and other movement disorders that are not uncommon. CEEG with video is useful to confirm the nonepileptic etiology to avert superfluous and potentially harmful treatment by excessive use of anti-seizure drugs (ASDs).

One final difficulty is the frequent occurrence of artifacts in ICU EEG that interfere with proper interpretation of CEEG. Some are common to all techniques using EEG but are more frequent in the critically ill patient. Some artifacts are specific to the ICU setting. These artifacts may exhibit rhythmicity or periodicity and require some expertise to be recognized and not mistaken for periodic brain activity or seizures.

GENERALIZED BACKGROUND ABNORMALITIES

Generalized background abnormalities are common in ICU EEG recordings and indicate diffuse or multifocal cerebral dysfunction affecting the gray and/or white matter. These abnormalities are nonspecific and are encountered in a variety of toxic-metabolic and structural processes. Structural processes causing generalized abnormalities in the EEG may be diffuse (e.g., widespread traumatic axonal damage or ischemic injury), focal with secondary generalized cerebral dysfunction (e.g., increased intracranial pressure from a space-occupying lesion or upper brainstem lesion with disruption of ascending pathways to the cortex), and appear multifocal.

Severity scales have been proposed that correlate EEG findings with clinical findings and prognosis after anoxic brain injury, or during hepatic or septic encephalopathy. One common classification scheme is described below and includes a clinical correlation:

Grade 1 (corresponds to a mild degree of encephalopathy):
- The predominant posterior dominant rhythm lies in the alpha frequency range and is regular and reactive, with intermittent theta activity;

Grade 2 (corresponds to a mild to moderate degree of encephalopathy):
- The posterior dominant rhythm is predominantly theta activity that is often reactive and which may be accompanied by alpha and/or intermittent delta activity;

Grade 3 (corresponds to moderate and moderate to severe degrees of encephalopathy):
- The background activity is predominantly delta activity. In this case, the presence of reactivity* and a higher amplitude carries a more favorable prognosis, whereas the absence of reactivity, lower amplitude, and presence of periods of attenuation (discontinuity) are less favorable.

OR
- Spindle coma* is present.

Grade 4 (corresponds to a severe degree of encephalopathy):
- Burst-suppression,

OR
- Alpha coma, beta coma or theta coma,

(Continued)

OR
- Diffuse attenuation (all activity less than 20 μV)

Grade 5:
- Electrocerebral inactivity

---

* Patients with nonreactive continuous generalized delta activity or spindles are usually comatose (i.e., they have a severe degree of encephalopathy) but their prognosis tends to be better than patients with Grade 4 EEG findings.

Source: Synek VM. Prognostically important EEG coma patterns in diffuse anoxic and traumatic encephalopathies in adults. *J Clin Neurophysiol*. 1988;5(2):161–174.

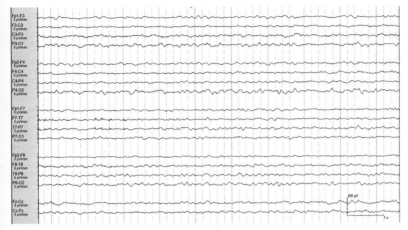

FIGURE 7.1. This is the EEG of a 59-year-old male with sepsis from a respiratory infection. The background is abnormal due to the absence of posterior dominant rhythm and the presence of continuous generalized polymorphic theta activity.

Generalized polymorphic slowing is characterized by the disappearance of normal fast EEG activity (alpha and beta), which is replaced by generalized polymorphic slow (theta and/or delta) activity. This indicates diffuse or multifocal cerebral dysfunction, typically involving the subcortical white matter, though is a nonspecific finding. Clinical correlates range from subtle alteration of mental status to stupor (see Chapter 2).

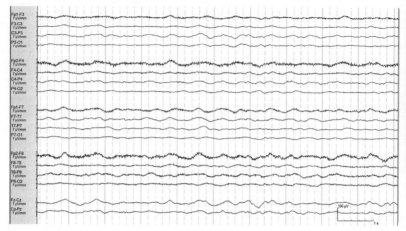

FIGURE 7.2. This is an example of generalized polymorphic 1 to 2 Hz delta activity on EEG recorded from a 55-year-old male with acute renal failure.

In the situation where an EEG contains generalized slowing, indicators of greater severity include pronounced low frequencies (delta vs. theta), poor variability, poor reactivity, low amplitude, and periods of attenuation. It should be remembered that the EEG indicates the degree of dysfunction at a given moment, and its prognostic value is dependent on the reversibility of the underlying disorder.

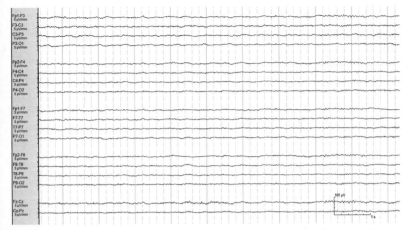

FIGURE 7.3. This is a low voltage (less than 20 µV) EEG in a 33-year-old female with fulminant hepatitis.

Diffuse attenuation consists of widespread low voltage electrocerebral activity. It is defined as all or most activity lower than 20 µV that is measured peak to peak, in a standard longitudinal bipolar montage. Typically, most or all of the activity is delta frequency that is often poorly reactive. This is a nonspecific finding that indicates severe global brain dysfunction, including the cortex diffusely, often due to anoxic injury or toxic, metabolic, ischemic, and inflammatory-infectious encephalopathies.

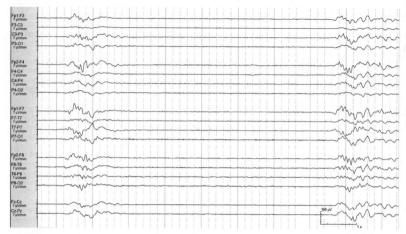

FIGURE 7.4. This EEG shows a burst-suppression pattern in a 62-year-old female after cardiac arrest. Bursts consist of theta and delta activity admixed with low voltage faster activity and rare epileptiform discharges. No clear cerebral activity is visible during the interburst interval.

In burst-suppression, periods of voltage attenuation (10–20 µV) or suppression (less than 10 µV), termed interburst intervals, alternate with bursts of activity. The bursts are variable but typically consist of high voltage delta/theta activity admixed with (poly)spikes/sharp waves. Burst-suppression is the manifestation of severe brain dysfunction, though sedation can also cause this pattern, especially with the use of barbiturates and propofol.

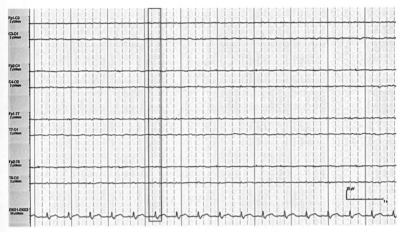

FIGURE 7.5. The absence of clear cerebral activity that is greater than 2 μV (electrical cerebral inactivity) in a 64-year-old female after cardiac arrest. Note the double distance montage and the high sensitivity (1 μV/mm) that magnifies the EKG artifact (box).

Electro-cerebral inactivity (ECI) is defined as the absence of cerebral activity on a carefully performed EEG using an ECI protocol. The assessment of ECI for the diagnosis of brain death requires a very specific protocol, including reading EEG at high sensitivity (2 μV/mm), using a double distance montage (inter-electrode distance ≥ 10 cm), and maintaining electrode impedances between 100 and 10,000 Ohms. There is a risk of amplifying artifacts in the EMG, EKG, etc. that should not be misinterpreted as brain rhythms. For use as an adjunctive test for the determination of brain death, all reversible causes of ECI should be excluded, including high doses of sedating medications, hypothermia, and marked metabolic dysfunction. The prognosis associated with ECI is mainly determined by the underlying etiology. It is invariably poor in predicting the outcome in a case of post-anoxic encephalopathy, but is less so in cases of drug overdose, toxic-metabolic encephalopathy, and severe hypothermia where the cause may have a reversible component.

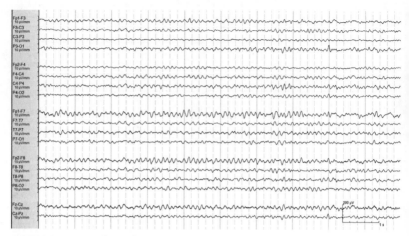

FIGURE 7.6. Frontally-predominant continuous alpha activity is present on EEG in a 58-year-old male in postanoxic coma (alpha coma). The alpha activity was not modified by stimulation.

Alpha coma is a unique and striking EEG pattern characterized by the presence of widespread prominent activity in the alpha frequency range. Unlike a normal alpha rhythm, the alpha rhythm in alpha coma has an anterior (frontal) predominance and displays no or minimal reactivity to stimulation. It is most commonly seen in postanoxic encephalopathy and with lesions of the middle to upper brainstem. Alpha coma typically indicates a poor prognosis, when it is due to anoxia, though it may have an independent predictive value when the clinical course and etiology is taken into account. For example, it may be encountered in severe toxic or metabolic encephalopathy and has a much better prognosis in these situations. At times, reactivity is preserved and this carries a more favorable prognosis. There are variants of alpha coma, with similar significance, where the rhythmic activity lies in the theta or beta range (termed theta and beta coma). All three forms may coexist in the same patient.

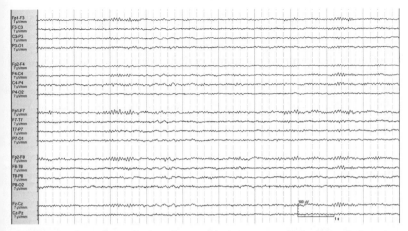

FIGURE 7.7. Frontally-predominant beta activity is present on EEG with a spindle-appearing morphology in a 36-year-old male in coma after a midbrain hemorrhage (spindle coma).

Spindle coma denotes the association of coma with EEG features that resemble N2 sleep. It is another form of rhythmic coma similar to alpha coma in which the background consists of prominent poorly reactive low-voltage beta activity that resembles sleep spindles. It is seen with traumatic and atraumatic etiologies similar to those identified in patients with alpha coma, though spindle coma tends to carry overall a more favorable prognosis.

PERIODIC AND RHYTHMIC DISCHARGES

Up to 20% of critical care EEG recordings will show the presence of repetitive waveforms that recur with a nearly periodic regularity. These discharges include periodic (sometimes epileptiform) discharges (PDs). Between PDs the background may remain visible signifying an inter-discharge interval. Alternatively, rhythmic discharges may occur continuously where successive waveforms prevent identification of an inter-discharge interval.

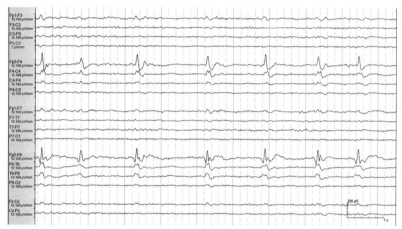

FIGURE 7.8. The EEG in a 65-year-old female with a subarachnoid hemorrhage and clipping of an aneurysm of the right middle cerebral artery. Note the 0.5 to 1 Hz right frontopolar LPDs with a diphasic/triphasic sharp morphology that followed an episode of nonconvulsive SE.

Lateralized periodic discharges (formerly known as PLEDs) usually reflect the presence of an acute (or subacute) focal brain lesion, though may reappear with acute reactivation of a chronic lesion. LPDs are most commonly associated with cerebral infarction, though intracranial hemorrhage, brain tumor or infection may act as predisposing etiologies. They may also rarely follow seizures in the absence of a structural lesion. They are transient and usually disappear after a few days to two weeks and rarely may be persistent.

Patients with LPDs often display impaired consciousness and focal neurological signs and between 50% and 90% of them will manifest seizures during the acute phase of their illness.

LPDs are usually felt to represent an interictal pattern. However, they may be occasionally associated with transient clinical manifestations, including time-locked motor features such as clonic jerks where they represent a form of focal SE.

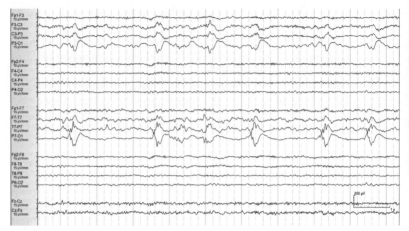

FIGURE 7.9. 0.5 to 1 Hz left posterior LPDs with low voltage sharp fast rhythm (LPDs+) in a 67-year-old male with a glioblastoma.

LPDs may appear as spikes, sharp waves, sharply contoured or blunt delta waves, and spike-and-wave complexes, repeating at periodic or nearly periodic intervals.

When associated with focal rhythmic fast (sometimes called transitional) activity or superimposed rhythmic delta, they are called LPDs+ (fka "PLEDs plus") as opposed to LPDs proper (fka "PLEDs proper"). LPDs+ often alternate with or precede LPDs proper in the same individual and probably carry a higher risk of acute seizures and SE.

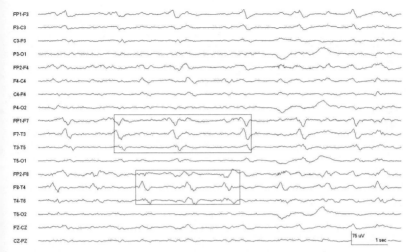

FIGURE 7.10. Bilateral independent periodic discharges (BIPDs) are present on EEG in a 75-year-old woman with postanoxic encephalopathy. The discharges occurred independently over the temporal regions (boxes).

In BIPDs, formerly known as bilateral independent periodic lateralized epileptiform discharges [BIPLEDs]), the discharges appear similar to LPDs, though are seen independently in both the hemispheres. They suggest a multifocal or commonly a global cerebral dysfunction. Patients with BIPDs are typically comatose. The risk of seizure associated with BIPDs is slightly lower than with LPDs (50%). The most common etiology is an anoxic-hypoxic injury, though stroke, central nervous system (CNS) infection, and toxic/metabolic/septic encephalopathies may occur.

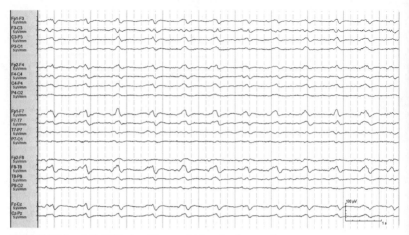

FIGURE 7.11. 1 Hz GPDs in a 44-year-old female after cardiac arrest.

GPDs, formerly known as Generalized Periodic Epileptiform Discharges (GPEDs), are bilateral synchronous symmetrical discharges. They are nonspecific and suggest diffuse cerebral gray matter dysfunction, as occurs with various toxic/metabolic etiologies (including sepsis), after anoxic injury, or in Creutzfeldt-Jakob disease. Consciousness is significantly disturbed in virtually all patients with GPDs. Seizures or SE occur in just under 50% of patients with GPDs. GPDs themselves may be an ictal pattern, including as an EEG correlate of nonconvulsive and myoclonic SE associated with postanoxic encephalopathy, especially when the frequency of the GPDs occur at 2 Hz or greater, or when they fluctuate or are evolving.

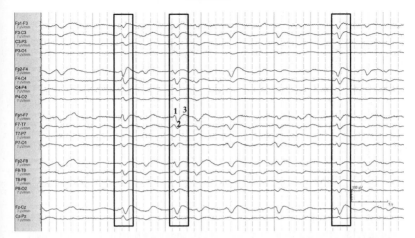

FIGURE 7.12. 0.5 to 1 Hz GPDs in a 64-year-old female with acute renal failure. Note the triphasic morphology present with some discharges (boxes). Triphasic waves have three phases; (1) an initial negative phase, (2) a prominent positive phase, and (3) a final negative phase. Note the increasing duration of the three phases (i.e., phase 3 is longer than phase 2, which is longer than phase 1). Phase 1 or phase 3 might be of small amplitude or absent and may mimic nonconvulsive status epilepticus (NCSE) when they are continuous.

GPDs vary in shape and include spikes, polyspikes, sharp waves, and sharply contoured slow waves. GPDs may sometimes have a triphasic morphology. Triphasic waves were initially thought to be specific markers of hepatic coma. However, they are now known to be nonspecific and may be encountered in a variety of toxic-metabolic-encephalopathies, neurodegenerative disorders (especially Creutzfeldt-Jakob Disease), and even occur during or following seizures and SE. Although differences between GPDs of epileptic and metabolic etiology exist at the population level, no single characteristic reliably allows their differentiation in a particular individual. While benzodiazepines are used as an initial treatment for seizures, it is important to note that both epileptic and metabolic GPDs may disappear after administration of an intravenous benzodiazepine.

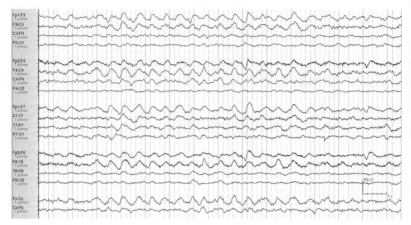

FIGURE 7.13. This is a 15-second epoch of EEG showing a burst of 1 to 2 Hz frontally predominant generalized rhythmic delta activity (GRDA) in a stuporous 55-year-old male with renal and hepatic failure.

Generalized rhythmic delta activity (GRDA) consists of bilateral symmetrical and synchronous monomorphic delta activity that is either seen diffusely or predominantly in the anterior regions. It can occur as brief intermittent runs (including frontal intermittent rhythmic delta activity [FIRDA]) or be continuous GRDA.

GRDA is a frequent pattern in critically ill individuals. Initially it was thought to indicate the presence of a deep midline lesion. It most commonly reflects a moderate degree of global cerebral dysfunction and is seen in a variety of toxic, metabolic, and postanoxic etiologies. It may also indicate the presence of a lesion involving the frontal lobes, especially when it is consistently asymmetric.

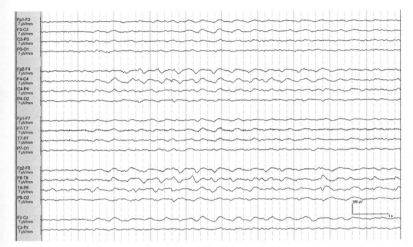

FIGURE 7.14. Right fronto-temporal lateralized rhythmic delta activity (LRDA) in a 22-year-old male with Mycoplasma pneumonia-related encephalitis.

Lateralized rhythmic delta activity (LRDA) consists of nonevolving runs of monomorphic delta activity with a focal or hemispheric distribution. In critically ill individuals, it usually indicates the presence of an acute focal brain lesion involving the cortex and/or the deep gray matter structures. In our experience, it carries a risk of seizures similar to that associated with LPDs (60%) and is in fact often encountered together with LPDs.

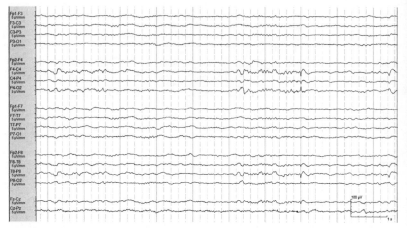

FIGURE 7.15. Two brief potentially ictal rhythmic discharges B(I)RDs in the right centro-parietal region in a 78-year-old male with a subdural hematoma who demonstrated NCSz on CEEG in the same region.

Brief potentially ictal rhythmic discharges B(I)RDs are rhythmic bursts of waves that share many characteristics with seizures (sharp morphology and/or evolution in frequency or morphology and/or field of spread), but last less than ten seconds. They have been primarily described in neonates with seizures, though may also occur in critically ill adults where they are almost always associated with clinically relevant (i.e., longer) seizures.

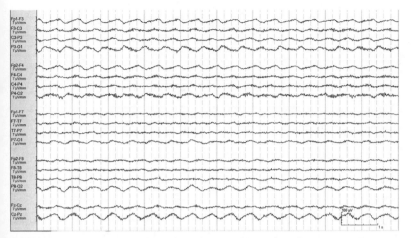

FIGURE 7.16. Continuous GRDA with superimposed low voltage beta activity. The "extreme delta brush" pattern was present in a 33-year-old female with anti-NMDA encephalitis.

Extreme delta brushes consist of prominent and prolonged (minutes to hours) runs of rhythmic delta activity (RDA), typically frontally maximal, with superimposed low voltage beta or gamma (30–40 Hz) activity. These complexes resemble the delta brushes of neonates, but are continuous or nearly so. They have been described in anti-NMDA encephalitis, especially with more severe cases. It is unclear if these complexes represent an ictal or interictal pattern, though eliminating them with treatment can be difficult and has not led to rapid improvement in most cases.

SEIZURES/STATUS

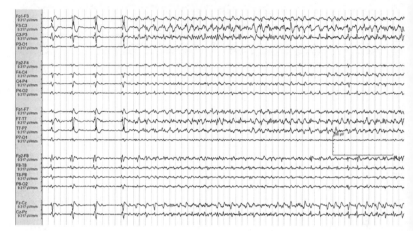

FIGURE 7.17. This is a 60-second epoch of EEG showing a left hemispheric seizure in 81-year-old male with Herpes Simplex Encephalitis 1(HSV1). Note the presence of left hemisphere LPDs and the ictal onset pattern consisting of sharply contoured 1 Hz delta activity with admixed faster activity and slow evolution. Evolution is best seen at a display speed that is faster than the conventional speed.

Seizures occur in 10% to 20% of critically ill patients undergoing CEEG. The majority of these (~75%) are nonconvulsive and require EEG to be detected. Risk factors include acute brain injury, sepsis, renal failure, coma, young age, and prior clinical seizures. Subtle motor manifestations may occur, including eye deviation, nystagmus, face or finger twitching. Ictal patterns on EEG that are seen in the ICU often differ from seizures in alert patients with chronic epilepsy. NCSz on the EEG have less distinct onset and offset, slower evolution, slower maximum frequencies, and typically occur on an abnormal background. All of these features make them harder to recognize. Evolving or fluctuating RDA, periodic discharges, and spike-and-wave complexes may all represent NCSz.

Using a longer time scale during EEG may allow better appreciation of the evolution of a slow rhythmic discharge.

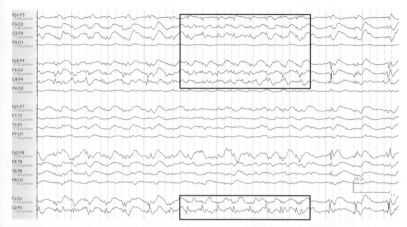

FIGURE 7.18. The EEG of a 71-year-old male that suffered a left frontal ischemic stroke following cardiac surgery with extracorporeal membrane oxygenation. The patient was obtunded and had intermittent twitching of the right hand. Note the presence of continuous 1 to 2 Hz rhythmic spike-and-wave complexes and poly-spike-and-wave complexes that are most prominent over the left frontal region alternating with runs of 2 to 3 Hz rhythmic sharp waves (box).

Almost half of the seizures encountered in the critically ill are SE. Like NCSz, SE is most often nonconvulsive in the ICU setting, occurring in patients with a severely impaired level of consciousness. Minor clinical manifestations, however, may be seen, including nystagmus, eye deviation, autonomic changes, repetitive eye opening, and subtle face or limb myoclonus.

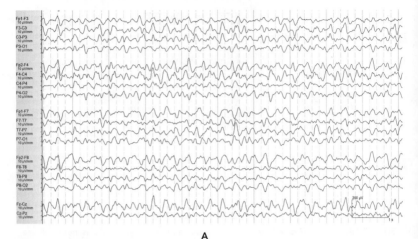

A

FIGURE 7.19. The EEG of a 75-year-old female with an intraparenchymal hemorrhage and coma. Note the presence of high amplitude sharply-contoured rhythmic activity at times reaching greater than 4 Hz. This pattern was ultimately felt to represent generalized NCSE. The patient received two boluses of lorazepam (total dose: 5 mg) with EEG improvement (B and C). She progressively regained consciousness over the next 24 hours.

Although criteria for NCSz and SE have been proposed, some patterns remain difficult to categorize and are thought to belong to a continuum that reflects a dynamic state between interictal and ictal activity.

When in doubt, the administration of a fast-acting ASD such as a benzodiazepine may help clarify the ictal nature. Electrographic *and* clinical improvements are both required to confirm the diagnosis of NCSE. A negative test devoid of electro-clinical resolution is inconclusive and does not exclude the diagnosis of NCSE. Clinical improvement may take up to 24 hours to be noticed.

(Continued)

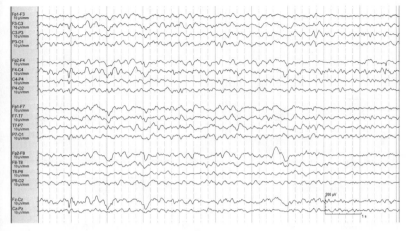

B

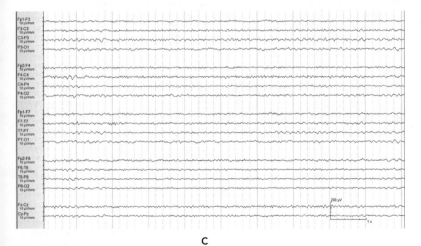

C

FIGURE 7.19. (*Continued*)

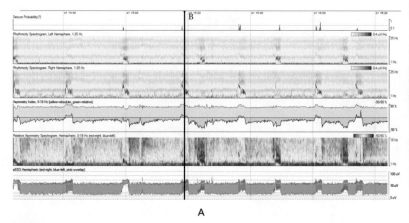

A

FIGURE 7.20. Quantitative EEG (A) in a 50 year-old female with invasive aspergillosis. Seizures are easily noticed on the rhythmicity spectrogram (rows 2 and 3) by the vertical marks in blue, on the asymmetry index in row 4 (upward deflection = right and downward deflection = left), and relative asymmetry spectrogram (row 5) showing relative power (red = right and blue = left). The duration of the epoch is 2 hours. The seizure periodicity is 20 minutes in the right hemisphere and 30 minutes in the left hemisphere.

Cyclic seizures are an uncommon form of SE encountered in critically ill patients in which discrete, usually brief, seizures occur with a nearly regular periodicity every 2 to 20 minute interval. The reasons for a cyclic pattern are poorly understood, but may include the transient efficacy of endogenous inhibitory mechanisms involved in seizure termination.

(Continued)

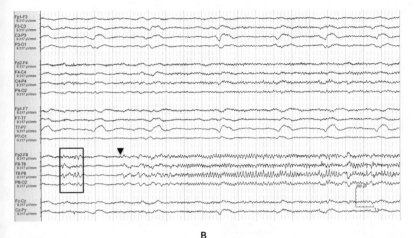

B

FIGURE 7.20. (*Continued*)   (B) This 20-second epoch of EEG shows a right temporal seizure (arrowhead). Note the presence of a B(I)RD 2 seconds before the seizure onset (box) and left hemispheric LPDs.

STIMULUS-INDUCED PATTERNS

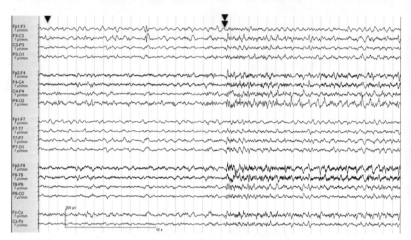

FIGURE 7.21. This 40-second page of compressed EEG is taken from a 60-year-old female with subarachnoid hemorrhage and left middle cerebral artery (MCA) vasospasm. Stimulation by nostril tickling (onset of stimulation indicated by arrowhead) is followed by the appearance of right posterior LPDs (onset indicated by double arrowhead).

In as many as 20% of comatose or stuporous patients undergoing CEEG periodic, rhythmic, or ictal-appearing discharges are consistently elicited by various kinds of non-noxious (noise, nursing) or noxious (nostril tickling) stimuli. Conversely, rhythmic and periodic patterns may also disappear upon arousal following stimulation, though this is much less common. The exact mechanism of stimulus sensitivity remains unclear, but probably implicates the combination of thalamocortical activation and cortical hyperexcitability.

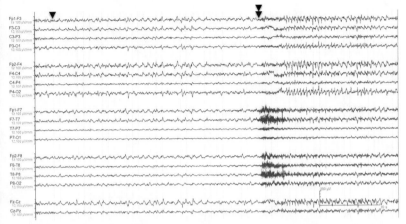

FIGURE 7.22. This 60-second epoch of EEG occurred in a 51-year-old female with a history of generalized epilepsy of unknown origin who was admitted for SE. Stimulation (due to a nurse replacing her IV line is indicated by an arrowhead) consistently elicited brief electro-clinical seizures (double arrowhead) manifest as runs of frontally predominant generalized fast activity with clinical features of myoclonic jerks mainly of the proximal lower limbs. This example represents stimulus-induced discharge with a clinical correlate.

Despite the classic EEG teaching that patterns induced by arousal are usually unrelated to seizures, it is clear that alerting stimuli are able to elicit ictal discharges that are sometimes associated with clinical manifestations. The presence of a clinical correlate likely depends on the involvement of the motor pathways and the ability of a discharge to propagate caudally from the cortex.

BRAIN MONITORING WITH QEEG

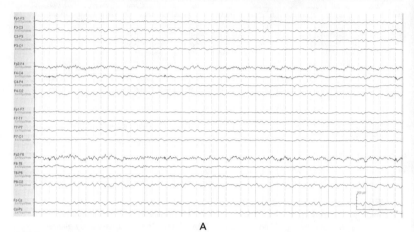

A

FIGURE 7.23A–D. This EEG represents a 63-year-old male with subarachnoid hemorrhage from a ruptured right anterior communicating artery aneurysm. (A) 10 seconds of EEG on day 2 after bleeding: the background consists of diffused symmetrical theta activity.

A decrease in brain perfusion is associated with progressive EEG changes that reflect the degree of ischemia:

Cerebral blood flow (mL/[100 g/min])	EEG correlate
25–35	Attenuation of alpha and beta activities
18–25	Polymorphic theta slowing
12–18	Polymorphic delta slowing
<10–12	Attenuation of all activities

(*Continued*)

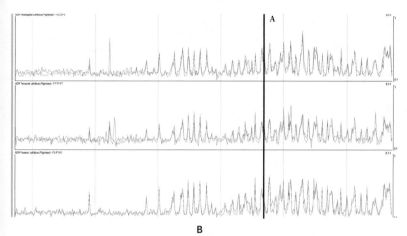

B

FIGURE 7.23. (*Continued*)   (B) Alpha-delta ratio values in the left (blue curves) and right (red curves) parasagittal (top), temporal (middle), and posterior (bottom) regions are symmetric and show strong variability prior to focal ischemia. The epoch of EEG in Figure 7.23 (A) is taken from segment A in Figure 7.23 (B).

These changes present on EEG reflect the corresponding functional changes of the brain that is produced when blood flow declines. This sequence of slowing and then attenuation is also reversible in the opposite direction when cerebral blood flow is maintained at a rate that is still adequate to perfuse the brain at a level that is above the threshold that exceeds that required to produce irreversible damage.

Thus, EEG provides a therapeutic window of opportunity to treat progressive ischemia before infarction ultimately occurs. Quantitative EEG analysis (using methods such as the Fourier transform) allows the computation of indices (alpha/delta ratio, relative alpha variability, symmetry measures) and their display as long-term trends to facilitate the detection of ischemic changes, which usually happen over long periods of time.

(*Continued*)

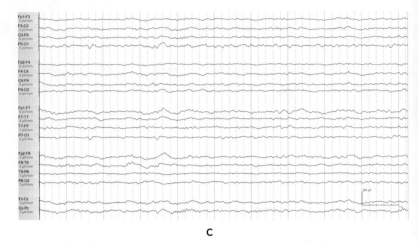

C

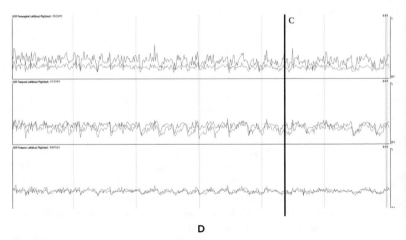

D

FIGURE 7.23. (*Continued*)   (C) 10 seconds of EEG on day 5 after bleeding: the background consists of generalized delta and theta activity. Low voltage fast activity is visible in the left fronto-central region but is attenuated in the right hemisphere. (D) Alpha-delta ratio values show less variability compared to day 2 and are lower over the right paracentral region. A CT angiogram demonstrated significant vasospasm of the right anterior cerebral artery.

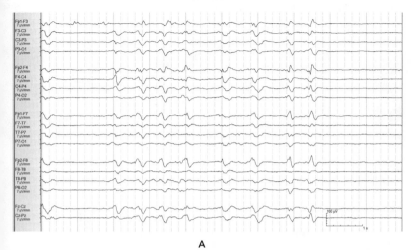

A

FIGURE 7.24 A–D. Continuous EEG monitoring was obtained during severe acidosis that progressively developed over hours in a 22-year-old patient with limbic encephalitis treated with high-dose midazolam and ketamine. Three noncontiguous 10-second EEG pages at 4 hour-intervals show a burst-suppression pattern in (A) with increasing duration of interburst intervals and shortening bursts in (B), and finally diffuse suppression in (C). (D) represents a total of 12 hours of quantitative EEG analysis.

In addition to ischemia, various pathophysiological processes are accompanied by EEG changes that can be quantified and displayed using QEEG analysis. Examples include raised intracranial pressure, systemic hypotension, acidosis, and the effect of medication.

(Continued)

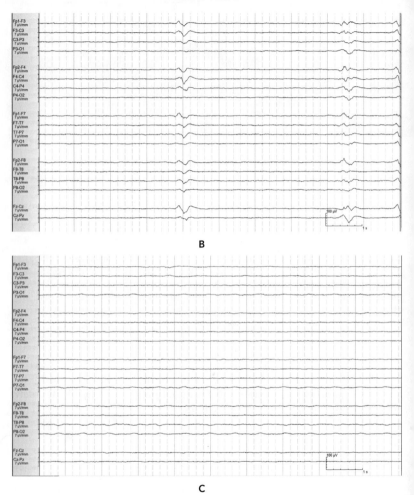

FIGURE 7.24. (*Continued*)

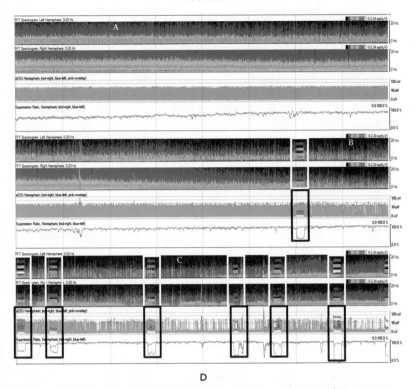

D

FIGURE 7.24D. (*Continued*)   Quantitative EEG analysis. From the top to bottom, a compressed spectral density array of the left and right hemisphere, amplitude-integrated EEG (aEEG) of left (blue) and right (red; superposition in pink) hemispheres, and suppression index (percentage of time the background amplitude is lower than a preset threshold that is typically 5 μV) of the left (blue) and right (red) hemisphere are represented by three successive 4-hour epochs. Note the progressive decrease in spectral power, the increase in discontinuity (aEEG trace) and the increase in suppression index. Oscillating bed artifacts are visible in all trends (boxes). Three EEG epochs that are shown in Figure 7.24 are represented by the letters A to C.

ARTIFACTS

The ICU is a hostile environment for EEG recording. Multiple sources of extra-cerebral signals exist and obtaining a study devoid of artifact is nearly impossible. Some well-known artifacts are common to all EEG recordings (EKG, eye movements, muscle activity, sweating, electrode instability, etc.) but prolonged recordings are more prone to technical issues than shorter ones.

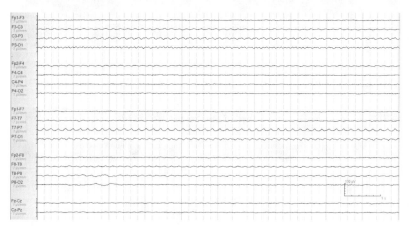

FIGURE 7.25. Oscillating bed artifact created 5 Hz sinusoidal activity. Although this activity may resemble physiologic theta in the ICU, notice the nonphysiologic field and the perfectly regular frequency.

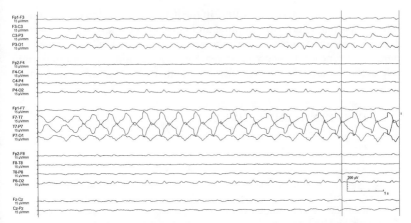

FIGURE 7.26. Rhythmic artifact seen on EEG occurred from chest compressions during cardiopulmonary resuscitation. Note the adjacent phase reversal of opposite polarity in channels 9 to 12 indicative of a nonphysiologic field.

The ICU environment is also characterized by the presence of specific signal generators that can produce peculiar artifacts that require some experience to recognize, such as mechanical ventilation (see Chapter 1), ventricular assist devices, oscillating beds, hemodialysis, and chest percussion. Recording video helps prevent error during interpretation of the EEG.

CHAPTER 7

Over the last two decades, EEG in the ICU has engendered tremendous interest. With advances in computer and network technology, it has become possible to continuously record and store video and EEG data over long periods of time, and review them remotely. CEEG now plays an important role in the management of critically ill patients with impaired mental status.

ADDITIONAL RESOURCES

Articles

Chong DJ, Hirsch LJ. Which EEG patterns warrant treatment in the critically ill? Reviewing the evidence for treatment of periodic epileptiform discharges and related patterns. *J Clin Neurophysiol.* April 2005;22(2):79-91.

Foreman B, Claassen J. Quantitative EEG for the detection of brain ischemia. *Crit Care.* March 20, 2012;16(2):216.

Foreman B, Claassen J, Abou Khaled K, et al. Generalized periodic discharges in the critically ill: a case-control study of 200 patients. *Neurology.* November 6, 2012;79(19):1951-1960.

Friedman D, Claassen J, Hirsch LJ. Continuous electroencephalogram monitoring in the intensive care unit. *Anesth Analg.* August 2009;109(2):506-523 [2009 ed.].

Friedman DE, Schevon C, Emerson RG, Hirsch LJ. Cyclic electrographic seizures in critically ill patients. *Epilepsia.* February 2008;49(2):281-287.

Gaspard, N, Manganas, L, Rampal, N, Petroff, OAC & Hirsch, LJ. Similarity of Lateralized Rhythmic Delta Activity to Periodic Lateralized Epileptiform Discharges in Critically Ill Patients. *JAMA Neurol.* 2013;70(10):1288-1295.

Hirsch LJ, Laroche SM, Gaspard N, et al. American Clinical Neurophysiology Society's Standardized Critical Care EEG Terminology: 2012 version. *J Clin Neurophysiol.* February 2013;30(1):1-27.

Hirsch LJ, Claassen J, Mayer SA, Emerson RG. Stimulus-induced rhythmic, periodic, or ictal discharges (SIRPIDs): a common EEG phenomenon in the critically ill. *Epilepsia.* February 2004;45(2):109-123.

Hirsch LJ, Pang T, Claassen J, et al. Focal motor seizures induced by alerting stimuli in critically ill patients. *Epilepsia.* June 2008;49(6):968-973.

Hughes JR. Periodic lateralized epileptiform discharges: do they represent an ictal pattern requiring treatment? *Epilepsy Behav.* July 1, 2010;18(3):162-165 [Elsevier Inc].

Kaplan PW, Rossetti AO. EEG patterns and imaging correlations in encephalopathy: encephalopathy part II. *J Clin Neurophysiol.* June 2011;28(3):233-251.

Parsons-Smith BG, Summerskill WH, Dawson AM, Sherlock S. The electroencephalo-graph in liver disease. *Lancet*. November 2, 1957;273(7001):867-871.

Schmitt SE, Pargeon K, Frechette ES, Hirsch LJ, Dalmau J, Friedman D. Extreme delta brush: a unique EEG pattern in adults with anti-NMDA receptor encephalitis. *Neurology*. September 11, 2012;79(11):1094-1100.

Synek VM. Prognostically important EEG coma patterns in diffuse anoxic and trau-matic encephalopathies in adults. *J Clin Neurophysiol*. April 1988;5(2):161-174.

Yoo JY, Rampal N, Petroff OA, Hirsch LJ and Gaspard N. Brief Potentially Ictal Rhythmic Discharges (B(I)RDs) in critically ill adults. *JAMA Neurol*. In press.

Books

Hirsch LJ, Brenner RP. *Atlas of EEG in Critical Care*. 1st ed. West Sussex, UK: Wiley-Blackwell 2009:1-348.

LaRoche SM. *Handbook of ICU EEG Monitoring*. 1st ed. New York, NY: Demos Medical 2012:1-352.

8

Polysomnography

Bradley V. Vaughn and Will Underwood

Sleep is a reversible physiological state of decreased responsiveness. As a function of the brain, sleep is expressed by a variety of physiological manifestations. These manifestations represent the output of sleep, but not the core drivers for sleep. Sleep can be quantified by several methods. The most common method is direct observation, but today polysomnography utilizes multiple measures to evaluate the sleep state.

For over a century, the study of sleep has been directed toward understanding sleep as an active process. Loomis, in 1937, showed the electroencephalographic changes we now correlate with non-rapid eye movement (NREM) sleep. Sixteen years later, Aserinsky and Kleitman identified the features of rapid eye movement (REM) sleep. Early study of normal physiological processes led researchers in the 1960s to begin to study patients with disordered sleep.

In 1968, Rechtshaffen and Kales developed a manual that standardized the scoring of normal sleep for laboratories studying sleep in adults. This manual was recently replaced by the American Academy of Sleep Medicine (AASM) Manual for Scoring Sleep Stages and Associated Events in 2007 and was revised in 2012 and 2014 to categorize and quantify the sleep stages and associated events that remains the current standard.

POLYSOMNOGRAPHY AND TECHNIQUE

Polysomnography correlates three measures; brain electrical activity, eye movement, and muscle tone to define sleep stage. These parameters are only three of a much longer list of parameters that change with brain state, and thus the first important lesson for anyone interpreting polysomnography is to realize that these three parameters may not completely represent the brain state of sleep.

Electroencephalography (EEG)

As outlined in most of this text, EEG records the summation of the cortical neuronal synaptic electrical fields as a marker of brain activity (see Chapter 1). These fields are largely recordable due to the radial positioning of most synapses and encompass both thalamo-cortical and cortical-cortical networks. Accurate assessment of these electrical fields requires appropriate placement of electrodes and attention to the recording device. A minimum number of electrodes are placed according to the International 10–20 electrode placement system in the F3, F4, C3, C4, O1, O2, M1, and M2 positions (M = mastoid). The AASM recommends sampling EEG at 500 Hz (200 Hz minimum) with a 12 to 16 bit registry length for the analogue to digital converter. The AASM recommends that EEG signals are filtered by bandwidths of 0.3 to 35 Hz. However, the authors use a bandwidth of 0.3 to 70 Hz, avoiding the 60 Hz notch filter. They find that by including these bandwidths it allows for the interpreter to recognize 60 Hz artifact, which is important in determining electrical integrity of the recording.

Electrooculogram

Eye movements aid in determining the continuum of wakefulness to light sleep and reflects the hallmark of Stage R with REMs. The eye has a relatively strong electropositive charge on the cornea which allows for relatively easy detection of eye movements by measurement of the electrical field.

Electrodes may be placed just beyond each outer canthus. Typically, the left ocular (LOC) electrode is placed 1 cm below the horizontal midline, and the right ocular (ROC) electrode is placed 1 cm above the right eye. Both electrodes are then referenced to an ipsilateral inactive electrode such as the mastoid electrode. This montage makes vertical and lateral movements identifiable as waveforms of opposite phase or polarity. Alternatively, each outer canthus electrode (LOC and ROC) placed 1 cm below the horizontal midline may be referenced to the midline frontal polar electrode. This montage shows lateral movements as out of phase and vertical as in phase waveforms providing clearer identification of vertical eye movements. Sampling rates and bandwidths used for the electrooculogram (EOG) are similar to the parameters for EEG. Eye movements are designated as either rapid or slow eye movements based upon the speed of the initial electrographic deflection. Waveforms that are greater than 500 msec from the initial deflection to the first peak are defined as slow eye movements.

Submental Electromyogram

The muscle tone is the third parameter in determining sleep stages. Submental muscle tone diminishes gradually with depth of sleep in NREM sleep and is normally at the lowest point during REM sleep. Muscle tone is recorded by two surface electrodes placed 2 cm below the inferior edge of the mandible and 2 cm to the right and left of midline. The electrodes are referenced to an electrode placed in the midline 1 cm above the inferior edge of the mandible. Electrodes may be attached with collodion or paste and secured with tape. Sampling rates should be at 500 Hz with a display bandwidth of 10 to 100Hz.

Breathing and Respiration

Our breathing pattern and respiratory responses are influenced by the stage of sleep. Light sleep is associated with mild periodic breathing, whereas Stage N3 has very regular respiration. Stage R sleep is associated with the greatest variability. During sleep, our normal physiologic response to a low oxygen level and an elevated carbon dioxide level is altered and the capacity to compensate for them may be reduced.

Measurements of respiratory function must reflect the dynamic features of air flow, ventilatory effort, and respiratory function. Air flow indicates the movement of air in and out of the chest cavity and is reflected by measures of temperature, pressure, and CO_2 concentration ($[CO_2]$). Ventilatory effort is assessed by movement of the chest and diaphragm representing the intrathoracic pressure changes induced by breathing. Respiratory function is reflected by the concentrations of oxygen and carbon dioxide measurements. The parameters of air flow and ventilator effort are sampled at a rate of 100Hz with filter settings of 0.1 to 15 Hz.

Respiratory Flow

Standard polysomnography uses air temperature and nasal pressure as estimates of flow. Air temperature is a sensitive measure of respiratory airflow. Upon inspiration, air enters the body at room temperature and exits during expiration near body temperature. These temperature differences can be easily measured using a thermistor or thermocouple. The thermocouple is very sensitive to minor air flow and is best used to determine apneas. However, due to their sensitivity, they are poor at detecting partial flow restrictions. Air pressure is another mechanism to estimate airflow that is measured by a piezoelectric pressure sensor placed at the entrance of the nares. These devices are very sensitive to hypopneas, but do not detect very low airflow and, thus, are not the primary parameter for detection of apnea. Therefore it is the combination of the two airflow sensors that allows the clinician to accurately assess hypopneas and apneas.

Turbulence is an important feature of compromised airflow. Snoring produces turbulent air flow. Detection may be accomplished by a variety of mechanisms that detect the high frequency oscillations of turbulent airflow. Nasal pressure can detect snoring. Altering the parameters (sampling rate of 500 Hz and filters of 10 to 100 Hz) will identify these higher frequency bandwidths. Other devices may sound or measure vibration to reflect turbulence.

Respiratory Effort

The current gold standard for effort is to measure the intrathoracic pressure monitoring during respiration, though techniques are invasive and may disturb habitual sleep patterns. Alternatively, calibrated inductance plethysmography can quantitatively estimate chest and abdominal movement. Inductance plethysmography utilizes wire coils to generate and measure a change in the electromagnetic field produced by respiration. However, these sensors become uncalibrated upon movement, limiting their quantitative usefulness. Surface intercostal electromyography (EMG), electrodes placed over the fifth to eighth lateral intercostal space, may qualitatively assess the respiratory effort. Placing these electrodes in the inferior aspect of the rib cage permits identification of both diaphragmatic and intercostal activity. Alternative measures using piezoelectrodes and strain gauges are not recommended.

Respiratory Function

Respiratory function is measured by the exchange of oxygen and carbon dioxide. Oxygen levels are measured via a pulse oximeter. This device depends upon a clean connection to the epidermis and results may be skewed by motion, skin pigmentation, and finger nail polish or discoloration. Oximeters are typically placed upon pulsating tissue such as the finger or less commonly the ear lobe. The device should have a signal average time of no more than 3 seconds. Carbon dioxide levels can be estimated by continuous end tidal sampling or measured transcutaneously. For end tidal CO_2, a small tube connected to an infrared CO_2 detection unit is placed at the entrance of the nares.

Cardiac Monitoring

Assessment of cardiac function is reflected by measurement of the electrocardiogram (EKG). The EKG is represented by a modified Lead II electrode placement. Additional electrodes may be placed to delineate specific types of dysrhythmias.

Movement

Sleep is a time of relatively limited movement. Movement is represented by surface EMG. The arms and legs are sampled to represent movement. Electrodes are placed no more than 3 cm apart over the anterior tibialis muscles on each leg and over the brachioradialis or wrist extensors of the arms. The electrodes should have impedances below 10K Ohms and preferably under 5K Ohms with signal sampling and display similar to parameters used for submental and respiratory EMG.

Body position may potentially impact the development of respiratory events. Body position can be recorded by the technologist or measured by a position sensor. While position sensors can aid in denoting position, they are sometimes inaccurate and should be used in conjunction with direct observation by the technologist.

Behavior Monitoring

Behaviors are best recorded with time synchronized audio and video recording. Current standard infrared video cameras for night-time recording provide excellent quality images. Patients do not perceive the infrared light sources, but allows the viewer to see detailed movement and behaviors. The continuous audiovisual recordings should be time-linked to the polysomnogram (PSG) and is extremely helpful in linking physiological data with discrete behaviors and detecting other events such as detection of mask leaks.

The combination of the EEG, EOG, and chin EMG activity provides the basis for sleep stage scoring. The interpreter should score the stage of sleep that is best represented by a 30 second epoch. Wakefulness (Stage W) is determined by the presence of a posterior dominant rhythm, the presence of eye movements, and continuous muscle tone (Figure 8.3). Stage N1 is associated with a loss of the posterior dominant rhythm and slowing of the background to the theta bandwidth (Figure 8.4). Stage N2 is characterized by sleep spindles and K complexes (Figure 8.5) and Stage N3 is hallmarked by 0.5 to 2.0Hz, 75 µV slow waves occupying at least 20% of the epoch (Figure 8.7). Stage R, REM sleep, has a low fast frequency EEG, the presence of REMs, and atonia (Figure 8.8). Arousals are noted by a return of the baseline posterior dominant rhythm for at least 3 seconds during NREM sleep (Figure 8.12), and an increase in the chin EMG during Stage R.

At the start of every PSG, the technologist asks the patient to perform various tasks such as eye blinking, breath holding, moving their legs to test the integrity and obtain a baseline of the recording system. Additionally, the impedance of the recording electrodes is tested prior to each sleep study.

The terms below are commonly used in PSG:

1. Lights out: start of PSG
2. Lights on: end of PSG
3. Epoch – the amount of time (usually 30 seconds) in which the recording is staged for sleep.
4. Time in bed (TIB): total time spent by the patient in bed during the sleep study (including periods of wakefulness)
5. Total sleep time (TST): total time spent by the patient in bed during any stage of sleep
6. Sleep efficiency: (TST/TIB) × 100, expressed as percentage
7. Wakefulness after sleep onset (WASO): time spent awake after the first epoch of sleep and before final awakening
8. Sleep latency: time from lights out to the first epoch of sleep
9. REM latency: time from the first epoch of sleep to the first epoch of REM sleep
10. % Stages N1, N2, N3, R: (time spent in each stage/TST) × 100, expressed as a percentage

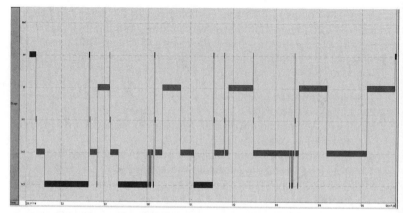

FIGURE 8.1. A hypnogram of a normal sleep cycle.

A hypnogram is a graph of the sleep stages over time. A hypnogram of normal subjects reveals sleep cycles through the night. The cycles of alternating NREM and REM sleep changes over the lifecycle. Sleep progresses throughout the night. The majority of Stage N3 (slow-wave) sleep is in the first third of the night while the majority of REM sleep is in the latter half of the night. This progression is indicative of two underlying forces that drive the sleep wake cycle: homeostatic drive and circadian drive. The homeostatic drive builds through the period of wakefulness and acts as a drive to enter sleep. Slow wave sleep appears to correlate with the decompression of this homeostatic drive. REM sleep appears to have a greater association with the core body temperature and, thus, a greater relationship to the circadian rhythm. The hypnogram eloquently illustrates the dynamic interplay of these two forces in sleep.

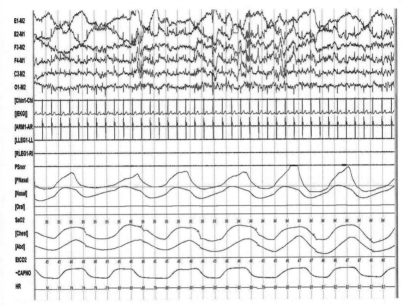

FIGURE 8.2. A 30-second page (epoch) of a PSG demonstrating the standard display montage.

In a routine PSG, many physiological parameters are recorded to determine the normal and abnormal features or stages of sleep. Physiological parameters commonly recorded are included in Figure 8.2; electroencephalogram (EEG) is represented on the channels labeled F3-M2, F4-M1, C3-M1, and O1-M2), submental electromyogram (EMG) (Chin), eye movements (electro-oculogram, EOG) (LOCLOC-M2, ROC-M2) to stage sleep. Additional parameters recorded include the heart rate [HR] digitally recorded by EKG or by pulse oximeter, and EMG activity from the arms [Arm1-Arm2] and legs (LLeg, RLeg). Respiratory flow is represented by measurements at the nose [nasal] by temperature and pressure and mouth [oral] by temperature, and the presence of snoring [Psnor]. Respiratory "effort" is a reflection of chest [chest] and abdominal [Abd] movement. Gas exchange is measured the downstream effect of oxygen saturation [SaO2] and end tidal CO2 [EtCo2]. End tidal CO2 also reflects the degree of respiratory flow measured by the digital readout of the "capnograph" [CAPNO]. Body position is evaluated with video and audio recording.

NORMAL SLEEP

Sleep is associated with a variety of physiological differences from awake. NREM sleep is characterized by relatively constant respiration, cardiac rhythm, and autonomic function. This is a state of relative quiescence and lower metabolic utilization. REM sleep, by contrast, demonstrates variation in respiration, cardiac function, and an absence of thermal regulation. Dreams are noted to occur in all stages of sleep. Dreams occurring in REM sleep are generally more vivid and more frequently recalled. Dreams occurring in non-REM sleep are generally poorly formed and less likely to be recalled.

Sleep changes through life and peaks in the newborn period. Sleep in this population is divided equally between REM and non-REM sleep. The infant cycles between the two states approximately every 40 minutes or faster. These cycles lengthen so that by the end of first year the cycles are approximately every 60 minutes compared to the adult period of 90 minutes. This first year is also filled with other developments. Spindles typically first appear between age 2 and 3 months and K complexes by 4 months. By the end of the first decade, sleep has developed its basic adult pattern, with REM sleep occurring approximately 25% of the sleep time. With advancing age, there is a decrease in the amplitude of slow waves and an increase fragmentation of the sleep due to spontaneous arousals. Daytime sleep also increases in the senior age group.

Staging Sleep

Staging of sleep follows rules that help categorize the conglomeration of the three parameters. Sleep recordings are divided into epochs. These epochs are typically 30 seconds long, however, in some research cases the epoch length may differ. Not uncommonly, there may be multiple features of different stages of sleep or wake within a single epoch. Despite the presence of multiple stages, each epoch is assigned the stage comprising the greatest portion of the epoch. This causes a smoothing of the sleep stages. Events such as arousals can be scored within epochs and will be discussed in the arousal section.

Scoring Stage W

Key Terms

Posterior dominant rhythm: A sinusoidal 8 to 13 Hz activity recorded over the occipital region with eye closure, attenuating with eye opening.

Eye blinks: Usually conjugate vertical eye movements at a frequency of 0.5 to 2 Hz present in wakefulness presenting as high amplitude positive polarity waveforms in the frontal and frontopolar regions.

REMs: Conjugate, irregular, sharply peaked eye movements with an initial deflection usually lasting less than 500 msec. These eye movements are seen in both Stage W and Stage R.

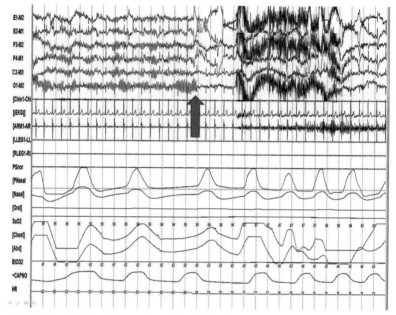

FIGURE 8.3. This is a 30-second epoch (displayed 30 mm/sec) demonstrating stage W. An alpha rhythm (posterior dominant rhythm) in the occipital channels (arrow) attenuates with opening of the eyes. Note the eye movements in the latter half of the epoch.

Stage W, or normal wakefulness, is often seen at the start of a PSG. Behaviorally, the subject should be able to interact with their environment. Characteristically, the features include the presence of the posterior dominant rhythm in the occipital regions, high tonic EMG activity, REMs, and irregular respiration. Occasionally, instead of a posterior dominant rhythm, low-voltage, mixed-frequency activity is seen, in which case the presence of eye blinks or REMs and high EMG activity would qualify the epoch to be staged as wake.

The posterior dominant rhythm in the occipital channels has a frequency of 10 Hz. With digital equipment, the clinician can view tracings at a variety of display windows (such as 10–12 seconds) to improve identification of EEG waveforms or slow the display window (3 minutes-30 seconds) to help identify slower frequencies (i.e., those associated with respiratory variation).

Stage N1

Key Terms

Slow eye movements: conjugate regular slow sinusoidal lower amplitude waveforms seen in the eye leads and fronto-temporal leads. These eye movements produce an initial deflection that last greater than 500 msec.

Vertex sharp wave (V waves): A monophasic sharply contoured wave with duration less than 0.5 seconds maximal over the central region and distinguishable from the background activity, but typically not large in amplitude.

The initial change in EEG between stage W and stage N1 is typically accompanied by loss of the posterior dominant rhythm, slow eye movements, and decrease in muscle tone. The transition may not occur as a "light switch" function, but a waxing and waning, as represented by the fragmentation of the alpha activity. Occipital electrodes are more sensitive in recording this fragmentation. As seen in Figure 8.4, the first sign of sleep onset is loss of alpha activity best seen in the O1-M2 and O2-M1 channels. At the same time, no significant change occurs in the C3-M2 channel.

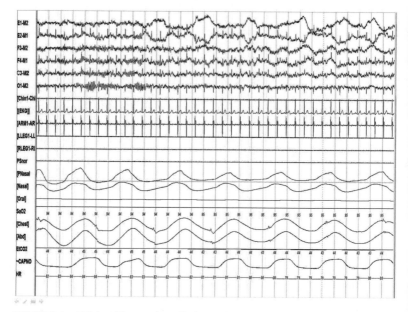

FIGURE 8.4. This is a 30-second epoch demonstrating stage N1 sleep with slow rolling eye movements. At the fifth and sixth seconds in this epoch, a posterior dominant rhythm can be seen, but subsequently attenuates.

Stage N1 sleep is the lightest stage of sleep and has the lowest threshold for arousal to wakefulness. Early in stage N1 sleep, the posterior dominant rhythm attenuates and the background activity slows in frequency involving a mixture of frequencies in the 4 to 7 Hz range. Slow rolling eye movements, as defined by the duration of upslope lasting longer than 500 msec, become more obvious and the chin EMG activity reduces from the high tone in wakefulness. Later in stage N1 sleep, vertex sharp waves may appear, but K complexes and sleep spindles are not present.

In this epoch of stage N1 sleep, the EEG consists of mixed-theta frequency activity and the minimal amount of slow eye movements. Central slowing and vertex sharp waves are present in the later stages of N1 sleep. Vertex sharp waves are surface-negative waves that are maximal in the central head region.

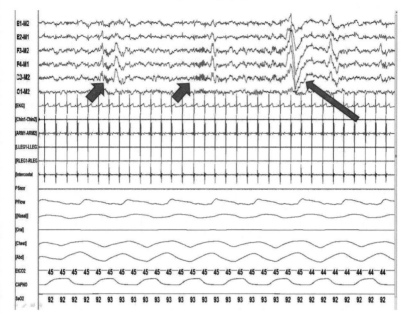

FIGURE 8.5. This is a 30-second epoch demonstrating stage N2 sleep with sleep spindles (short arrows) and K complexes (long arrow).

Stage N2

Key Terms

Sleep spindle: A train of sinusoidal waveforms with frequency between 11 and 16 Hz (12–14 Hz is most common) and a duration of ≥0.5 seconds. Sleep spindles are typically maximal in amplitude over the central head regions.

K complex: A well delineated diphasic waveform of negative sharp wave immediately followed by a positive sharp wave standing out from the background EEG with total duration ≥0.5 seconds, maximal in amplitude over the frontal regions.

(*Continued*)

The hallmark of stage N2 sleep is the presence of sleep spindles and K complexes. Sleep spindles consist of sinusoidal 11- to 16-Hz waveforms that last at least 0.5 seconds. K complexes consist of large diphasic waves with an initial negative sharp component followed by a positive component seen maximally expressed in the frontal electrodes. N2 sleep occurs whenever sleep spindles or K complexes occur without any intervening arousals or REMs and when it persists without proceeding to N3 or Stage R sleep. In the event a large movement occurs, if the movement is followed by a sleep spindle or K complex, the stage remains N2. If the movement is followed by slow eye movements, the stage following the movement reverts to Stage N1.

K complexes may occur in sustained sleep, but they also can occur as an evoked response to a stimulus. The K complexes associated with arousals are typically more broadly distributed in the frontal head region and have a more rounded appearance. These waveforms are differentiated from eye movements that have their maximal amplitude in the eye leads and not in the central head region and have out-of-phase deflections in the eye channels.

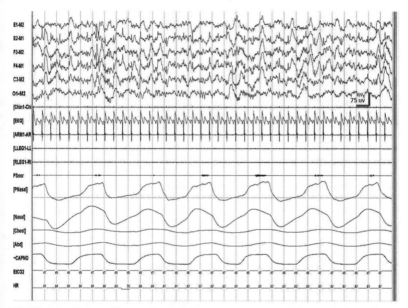

FIGURE 8.6. This is a 30-second epoch demonstrating stage N3 sleep with classic slow waves that comprise more than 20% of the epoch.

Stage N3

Key Term

Slow wave activity: Waves in the frequency of 0.5 to 2 Hz with a peak-to-peak amplitude greater than 75 µV measured in the F3-M2 or F4-M1 channels.

Stage N3 sleep is present when the EEG has 0.5 to 2 Hz slow waves that are greater than 75 µV and occupy at least 20% of the epoch. Sleep spindles, K complexes, and vertex waves may be present in this stage of sleep. Any nonpathological slow wave, including K complexes, are considered toward the 20% of slow wave activity in this stage. Stage N3 is also referred to as slow wave sleep (or slow sleep) due to the predominance of slow waves. However, the term Delta Sleep is a misnomer since the delta frequency includes waveforms that do not meet the slow wave criteria. High-amplitude slow waves are seen best in the F3-M2 and F4-M1 channels. Young individuals normally have higher amplitude slow waves than adults present in N3 sleep.

(Continued)

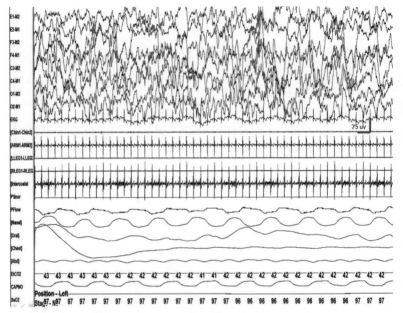

FIGURE 8.7. This is a 30-second epoch from a PSG that is taken from a child demonstrating stage N3 sleep.

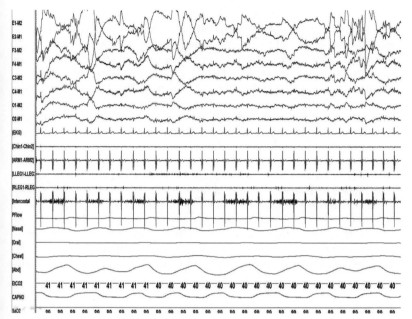

FIGURE 8.8. This is a 30-second epoch demonstrating stage R with frequent rapid eye movements (seen in EOG channels), lack of chin EMG activity, and mixed-frequency theta and alpha frequency EEG.

Stage R

Key Terms

Sawtooth waves: A train of sharply contoured or serrated, 2 to 6 Hz waves that are maximal in amplitude over the central or parietal head regions.

REMs: Conjugate, irregular, sharply peaked eye movements with an initial deflection usually lasting less than 500 msec. These eye movements are seen in both Stage W and Stage R.

Muscle Atonia: the loss of muscle tone as measured in the submental EMG.

(Continued)

Stage R is characterized by the appearance of REMs, low-amplitude, mixed-frequency EEG activity, and minimal chin EMG activity. The most characteristic feature of this stage is the presence of REMs. These are distinguished by their velocity. They typically have an initial deflection lasting less than 500 msec (some suggest less than 300 msec). These eye movements are out of phase deflections in the eye channels. This differentiates them from brain activity. The waveforms that occur in the EEG are commonly in the theta and alpha bandwidth. The EEG may also demonstrate a unique waveform known as sawtooth waves. These waves are typically in the central and parietal region and have the appearance as if a blade of a saw was turned upside down. These distinctive waves are a supportive feature of REM sleep but are not required for Stage R. Muscle atonia also distinguishes stage R. This feature is important because it signifies the inhibition of most of the skeletal muscles, sparing the diaphragm and a few other muscles. Occasional phasic EMG bursts may be seen, but these should be minimal and not involve the movement across a large joint. Physiologically, other changes also occur during Stage R. Blood pressure fluctuates, HR and respiration may become more irregular, and males develop penile tumescence in stage R.

(Continued)

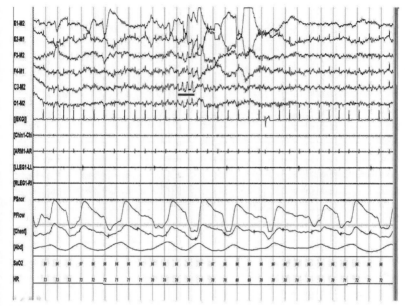

FIGURE 8.9. This is a 30-second epoch showing the start of stage REM and sawtooth waves as seen in the central head region.

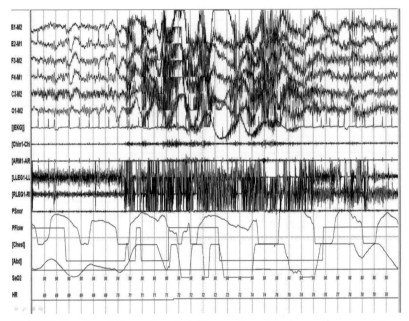

FIGURE 8.10. The middle portion of this 30-second epoch is obscured by movement. The movement is surrounded by alpha frequency activity indicating that the epoch should be scored as wake.

When an epoch contains movement, the presence of myogenic artifact may obscure the underlying EEG, EOG, and EMG. If it is preceded and followed by the same stage of sleep, it is scored as that stage of sleep. If the movement is greater than half of the epoch and alpha frequency activity is present (even if less than 15 seconds) or the epoch is immediately followed by wake, the epoch is scored as Stage W.

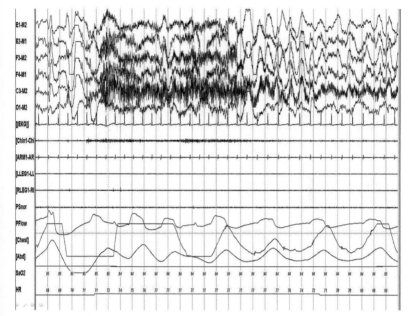

FIGURE 8.11. This 30-second epoch shows movement with slow wave preceding and following the movement. The epoch would be scored as Stage N3.

Staging Events

After the sleep/wake stage is determined, each epoch is then examined for other significant events which may include arousals, respiratory changes, movements, or cardiac phenomena. Each of these events forms their respective index to indicate their frequency and are typically represented by the number of events/TST spent in sleep per hour.

Arousals

Arousals are scored based upon an abrupt shift of state change. This may include the return of an alpha or theta frequencies (but not spindles) on arousal from NREM stages of sleep and last for more than 3 seconds. In Stage R, the change in the sleep stage must be accompanied by an increase in EMG activity. Arousals can only be identified/scored if there is at least 10 seconds of sustained sleep prior to the arousal. Arousals may be spontaneous or provoked. Arousals are classified based upon the cause. Arousals related to a respiratory event are known as respiratory related arousals. Limb movements are limb movement arousals. Those that are unclassified are identified as spontaneous arousals. Arousals are typically reported as a total number and as an index. The index is the total number of events divided by the amount of sleep in hours.

(*Continued*)

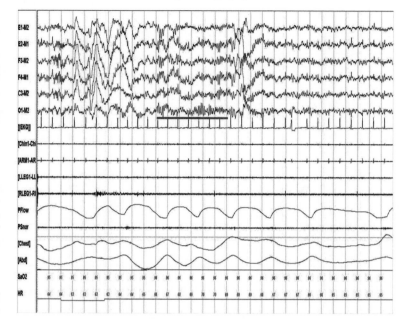

FIGURE 8.12. This 30-second epoch shows an arousal out of Stage N2 sleep. The faster frequencies in the EEG are underscored by the line. The arousal is not associated with an increase in EMG activity, but is preceded by a K complex. Note there are no clear slow eye movements following the arousal.

(Continued)

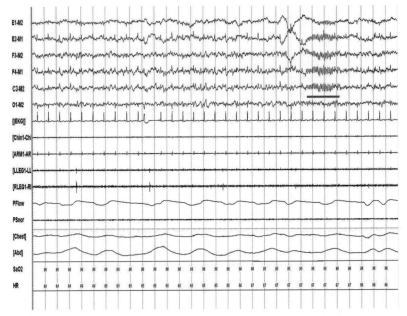

FIGURE 8.13. This 30-second epoch shows Stage R with a burst of alpha frequency activity. This activity would not be scored as an arousal since there is no increase in EMG activity to meet the requirements for an arousal from Stage R.

RESPIRATORY EVENTS

Key Terms

Apnea: Cessation of airflow ≥90% decrease in thermal sensor excursions compared to baseline for a minimum of 10 seconds in adults or for two respiratory cycles (breaths) in children. Apneas are classified as obstructive, mixed, or central based upon the respiratory effort.

Central apnea: the cessation of airflow (meeting the PSG) criteria for apnea unassociated with evidence of chest or abdominal movement (effort). In children these events must last greater than 20 seconds or last the equivalent of two breaths and be associated with a 3% desaturation or arousal.

Mixed apnea: the cessation of airflow lasting at least 10 seconds in adults or the equivalent of two breaths in children, initially unassociated with respiratory effort, but later demonstrating the presence of effort with chest or abdominal movement during the event.

Obstructive apnea: the cessation of airflow lasting at least 10 seconds in adults or the equivalent of two breaths in children associated with the presence of respiratory effort during the event.

Hypopnea: A common definition of hypopnea includes the reduction in airflow by 30% for at least 10 seconds in adults, or for two breaths in children accompanied by a ≥3% oxygen desaturation or occurring with an arousal. Hypopneas are best determined by using nasal pressure to measure flow.

Apnea hypopnea index: The total number of apneas and hypopneas divided by the number of hours of sleep.

Respiratory effort related arousal: A series of breaths characterized by increasing respiratory effort associated with evidence of flow limitation. Flow restriction may be represented by an inspiratory flattening in the nasal pressure (or positive airway pressure [PAP] device flow channel) or by an increase in end-tidal PCO_2 leading to an arousal from sleep. Respiratory effort related arousals have a minimum duration of ≥10 seconds in adults or the duration of at least two breaths in children.

(Continued)

Cheyne-Stokes breathing: A respiratory pattern with a crescendo-decrescendo phase accompanied by a change in breathing amplitude.

Hypoventilation: Increased PCO_2 concentrations of greater than 50 torr in adults (or greater than 52 torr in children) or a baseline elevation of PCO_2 concentrations during sleep of $\geq$10 torr exceeding 50 mmHg for a specified period of time.

PAP: This is forced airflow at a specific pressure to enhance the efficacy of respiration. PAP may be delivered at a constant pressure (CPAP) or at two separate pressures for inspiration and expiration (bi-PAP)

Respiratory changes demonstrate some variation based upon sleep stage. Breathing may be slightly irregular in Stage N1 and N2 but is quite regular in Stage N3. Stage R has the greatest variability overall, especially during periods of REMs. Breathing abnormalities include temporary absence of breathing (apnea), temporary reduction in breathing (hypopnea), periodic breathing, or breathing with a reduced/increased tidal volume (hypoventilation/hyperventilation). Because breathing cycles are much slower than EEG biorhythms, the use of a longer time base such as 60 to 240 seconds will permit delineation of certain respiratory patterns that might otherwise be difficult to detect.

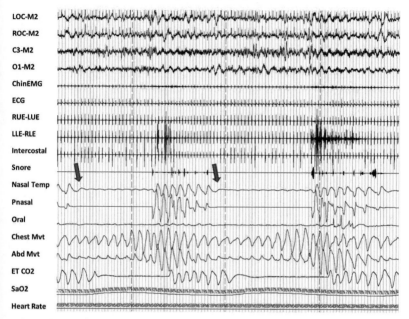

FIGURE 8.14. This is a 2-minute sample of a PSG that demonstrates two obstructive apneas (marked at their start by arrows). Despite the lack of airflow measured by the nasal temperature sensor, the abdominal and chest continue to move. Note the desaturations for each apnea are delayed because of the time of the blood involved to circulate to the peripheral oximeter on the finger. Also delayed is the signal for end tidal CO2 tracing. This is related to the length of the tube that samples air from the nose.

Apneas in adults must have a loss of greater than 90% of the airflow in the thermal sensor channels as compared to the pre-event baseline for a duration of at least 10 seconds. Apneas occur in three different forms: obstructive, central, and mixed apneas. Obstructive apneas have the presence of chest or abdominal movement throughout the event. These events are due to the collapse of the upper airway. During the event the abdominal and chest movement may shift out of phase to account for the lack of air flowing into the lungs. This *paradoxical movement* is a good clue to the obstructive nature of the event. These events are also associated with oxygen desaturation and arousals. The measured oxygen saturation may not drop for 20 seconds following the end of the apnea. This delay is related to the circulation time of blood traveling to the finger. Not uncommonly during the event, the HR may slow and rebound during the arousal. These events are also associated with a typical sound pattern, the abrupt stopping of snoring ending with a big gasp or snort. This characteristic sound is an important historical clue to the patient who may have obstructive sleep apnea (OSA).

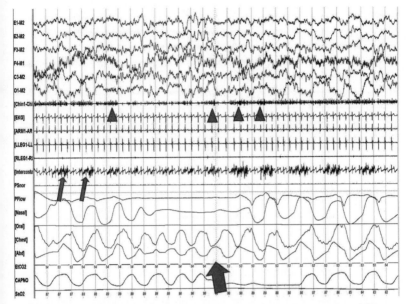

FIGURE 8.15. This 30-second epoch demonstrates an obstructive apnea in a child that has paradoxical movement of the abdomen and chest (thick arrow). This epoch also shows a good intercostals EMG (thin arrow) signal and snore artifact can be seen in the chin EMG (triangle). Apneas in children require two breaths to be scored as an apnea.

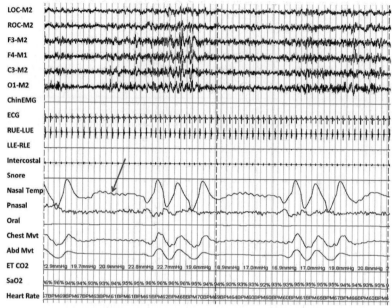

FIGURE 8.16. This 60-second epoch demonstrates central apneas. These events are characterized by the absence of airflow without compensatory movement in the chest and abdomen. The small deflections noted by the arrow indicate cardiobalistic movement of air that is captured in the nasal temperature channel. This indicates that the airway is patent. Also note similar movement is noted in the chest belt from direct cardiac movement.

Central apneas are scored when there is a cessation of airflow (for at least 10 seconds in adults) and no respiratory effort. This means that no compensatory movement is detected in the chest and abdominal belts, no electrical activity is noted in the intercostal EMG, and no evidence of pressure swings are noted in the intrathoracic pressure monitors. The presence of any of these would suggest obstruction. Central apneas in children must be 20 seconds or longer or be at least two breathing cycles in duration and be associated with a 3% oxygen desaturation or an arousal.

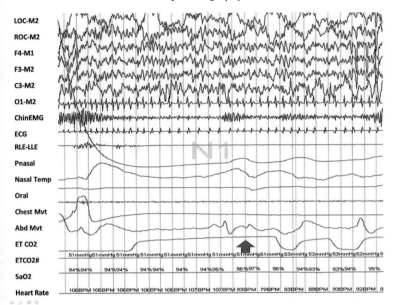

FIGURE 8.17. This 30 second epoch demonstrates a sigh or prolonged expiration. These are commonly confused with central apneas, but the feature of gradual increasing end tidal CO2 as marked by the arrow distinguishes this from an apnea.

Central apneas can occur in a variety of settings; at sleep onset, as a mixed obstructive apnea, in patients on narcotics, and during PAP titration. They also can be seen in patients with neurological disorders involving respiratory control, heart failure, at high altitudes, or with certain genetic anomalies. Measuring the concentration of carbon dioxide can help distinguish primary respiratory center failure (i.e., elevated EtCO2 seen as an effect from narcotics) from a secondary response of high CO2 apnea thresholds (e.g., Cheyne Stokes breathing). Sighs can look very similar to central apneas. Sighs are long exhalations and can be determined by recording the end tidal CO2. Sighs are normal phenomena (Figure 8.17).

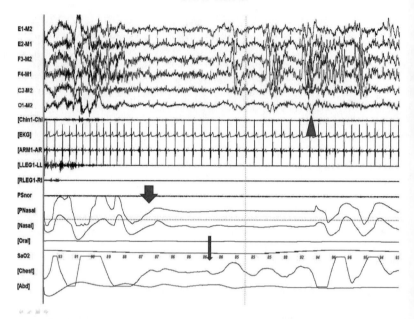

FIGURE 8.18. This 45-second epoch demonstrates the beginning of a mixed apnea. The short thick arrow shows the start of the apnea and the thin arrow shows the start of the chest movement. The time between the two arrows is the central apnea component. The time after the thin arrow is the obstructive portion of the apnea. Note the apnea ends and at the same time the arousal occurs (marked by the triangle).

Mixed apneas have a cessation of airflow with features of both central and obstructive apneas. These events start with no respiratory effort and then develop respiratory effort typically in the second half of the event. These events are also common in patients who have a mixture of central and obstructive apneas (Figure 8.18).

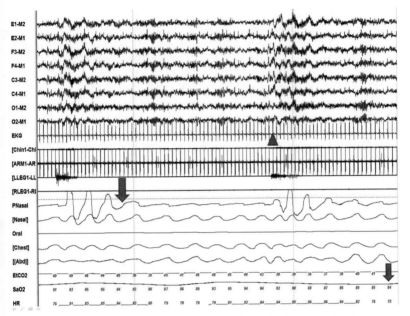

FIGURE 8.19. 60-second tracing demonstrates an obstructive hypopnea. The hypopnea lasts almost 30 seconds and is marked by a 50% decrease in the deflection of the nasal pressure channel. The thick arrow marks the start of the hypopnea with EMG activity in the intercostal muscles. The smaller arrow indicates the oxygen desaturation related to the hypopnea. The triangle marks the associated arousal.

Hypopneas are events with a partial reduction in airflow. The criteria for a hypopnea involves reduced respiration by greater than 30%, but less than a 90% decrease in baseline amplitude of the nasal pressure channel for at least 10 seconds in adults accompanied with an oxygen desaturation of at least 3%, or with an arousal. The physiological consequences of both apneas and hypopneas are thought to be the same, but apneas do not have the same requirement of being associated with either a desaturation or arousal in adults. In children, the hypopneas must last at least two breath lengths to be scored and must be associated with an arousal or oxygen desaturation of at least 3%.

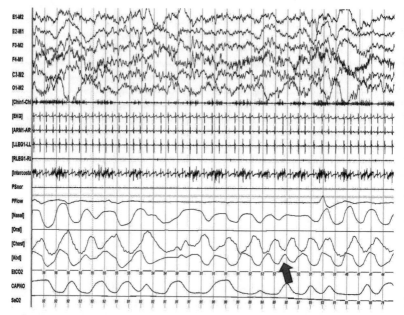

FIGURE 8.20. This is a 30-second epoch demonstrating an obstructive hypopnea associated with paradoxical motion of the chest and abdomen. This phase shift in the relationship of the waveforms is an important clue to obstruction of the upper airway, especially when other features may not be obvious.

Many clinicians use an index to determine the frequency and, therefore, the severity of the apneas and hypopneas. The Apnea-Hypopnea Index (AHI) is calculated as the total number of apneas plus hypopneas divided by the TST in hours. An AHI of less than 5 is considered normal for adults. Five to fifteen is considered mild, 15 to 30 is moderate, and an AHI of over 30 is severe. Some laboratories divide the AHI into obstructive and central. The obstructive AHI includes both obstructive and mixed events, whereas the central AHI contains only central events.

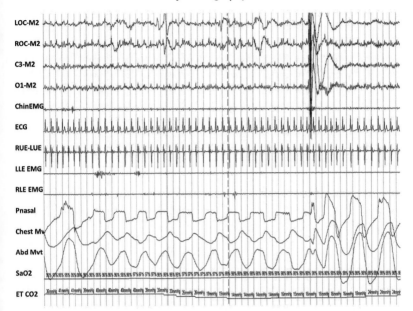

FIGURE 8.21. This 45-second window demonstrates a respiratory event-related arousal (RERA). This example shows flattening of the nasal pressure signal indicating flow limitation. In addition, you see the phase shift between the chest and abdominal movement so that it is out of phase during the RERA. This event could meet the criteria of a hypopnea, by the 2012 and 2014 criteria, if the reduction in flow is greater than 30% from the pre-event baseline.

Some obstructive respiratory events occur that are not hypopneas or apnea. These events are called respiratory event-related arousals (RERAs). They appear to cause arousals that are associated with flow limitation. The event can be associated with a progressive increase in snoring to reflect an increasing respiratory effort that is followed by an arousal. The events of flow limitation are noted by flattening of the inspiratory component of breathing in the nasal pressure channel. Clinically, there is loud snoring evident which is frequently associated with an arousal. Studies using esophageal pressure manometry show that these events are associated with an increase in negative intrathoracic pressure similar to that seen in apneas and hypopneas. The AASM suggests that these events be counted with obstructive apnea/hypopnea events. RERAs often resolve with continuous positive airway pressure (CPAP).

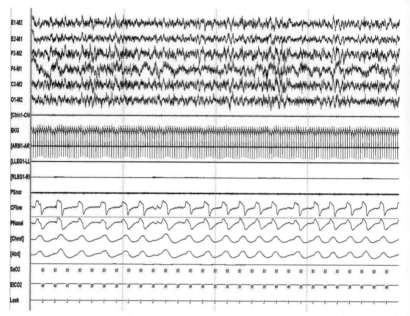

FIGURE 8.22. This is a 2-minute epoch demonstrating a patient with severe OSA that is being treated with CPAP.

Note the resolution of the apneas and desaturations upon treatment with CPAP.

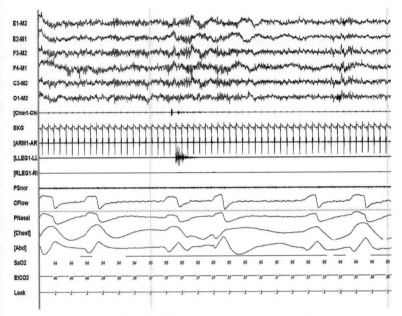

FIGURE 8.23. 60-second window demonstrates two central apneas in a patient undergoing CPAP titration for OSA syndrome.

Central apneas can emerge when patients with OSA undergo CPAP titration. The combination of obstructive apneas and treatment emergent central apneas has been termed complex sleep apnea. As the CPAP pressure is increased beyond the optimal range for the patient, central apneas may become more prominent. Some investigators have reported that these apneas improve with time, but some patients will need further respiratory support with bilevel PAP and ventilator assistance with adaptive servoventilation.

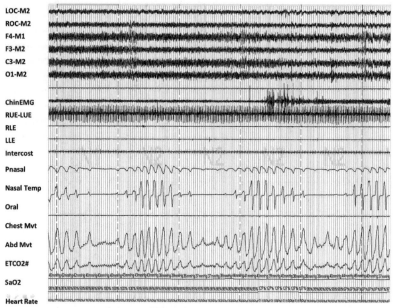

FIGURE 8.24. This is a 3-minute epoch that demonstrates Cheyne-Stokes respiration with periods of central apnea manifest as the absence of nasal/oral airflow and respiratory effort, alternating with periods of hyperpnea.

Cheyne-Stokes respiration is a cyclical pattern in which there is crescendo with subsequent decrescendo breathing between central apneas. This is usually seen in patients with congestive heart failure and central nervous system diseases affecting the brain. Apneas may be associated with an arousal or oxygen desaturation. These events differ from other apneas in that the arousals associated with Cheyne-Stokes respiration occurs during the peak of the hyperpnea and not at the termination of the apnea. Also, in patients with heart failure, the oxygen desaturation may be even later because of the greater circulation time. Occasionally obstructive components such as snoring may occur.

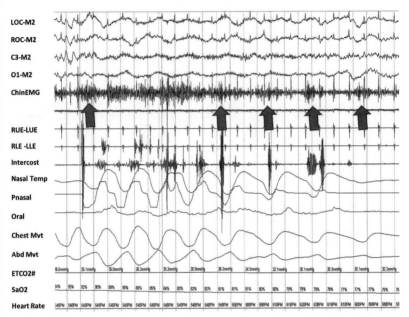

FIGURE 8.25. This is a 30-second epoch demonstrating snoring artifact in the Chin EMG channel. Note that the snoring artifact (arrows) matches the breathing rate.

Snoring can be a clue to airway compromise from narrowing of the primary respiratory tract during inspiration. This sound is the result of turbulent airflow causing tissues to vibrate. This vibration can be determined by several methods, including listening to the audio recording. In some laboratories, small microphones are placed at the supraclavicular notch, in others the nasal pressure is filtered to look at the faster frequencies consistent with sound waves. Snoring may also be detected as increase signal in the submental or chin EMG channel. During PAP titrations, the presence of snoring is an indication to increase the inspiratory pressure.

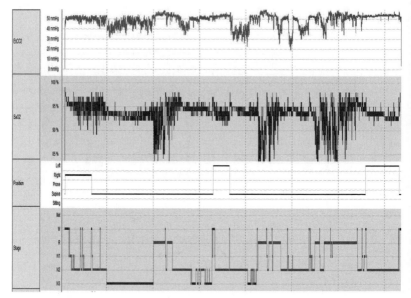

FIGURE 8.26. This is a hypnogram of obesity hypoventilation syndrome and demonstrates the value of measuring the end tidal CO2 levels through the night. The CO2 level is over 50 torr for more than 20% of the night with reduced oxygen saturation during periods of REM. This patient's overall AHI was 5.3 which is the hallmark of hypoventilation that is not due to apnea.

Hypoventilation that occurs during sleep can be detected by measuring CO2 levels. This is particularly important in individuals who are obese, with lung or neurological disease, or in children. Carbon dioxide levels can be measured in the nasal passage or transcutaneously. There are particular patterns of elevation. Obesity hypoventilation is characterized by normal CO2 levels in the standing position, but when patients are supine, their functional reserve capacity is compromised and the CO2 gradually rises. Obese individuals have the most trouble during Stage R sleep and may have severely prolonged oxygen desaturations during this time. Similarly, individuals with compromised diaphragmatic function, such as those with neuromuscular disease states, may have problems with Stage R sleep. An individual with lung disease can show a different pattern with an elevated CO2 level at the start of the study.

MOVEMENTS

Key Terms

Limb movements: These are defined by an increase in limb EMG activity that lasts for 0.5 to 10 seconds with voltage increases of 8 μV resolving to less than 2 μV above the resting state.

Periodic limb movements (PLMs): A series of at least four limb movements lasting at least 5 seconds but not greater than 90 seconds apart from the beginning of each single leg movement.

PLM index: The total number of PLMs during sleep divided by the total sleep in hours.

PLM arousal index: The total number of PLMs associated with arousals during sleep divided by the total sleep in hours.

Movements recorded from the legs and arms may normally occur during sleep. However, they may also occur during respiratory abnormalities. Some movements may impair sleep and subsequently result in daytime consequences. Unfortunately, the key elements that distinguish variations of normal physiologic limb movements from those that are pathological has not been clearly delineated.

Limb movements that occur during sleep most commonly appear in NREM sleep. The recording electrodes are placed on the anterior tibialis muscles in each leg and ideally the muscles of the arms should be included. For limb movements to be counted as significant, the event must meet the following criteria:

1. The duration of a limb movement event must be between 0.5 to 10 seconds.
2. The minimum amplitude of a limb movement event must be at least an 8 μV increase in EMG voltage above resting EMG.
3. The timing of the limb movement event is defined to begin at the point which there is an 8 μV increase in EMG voltage above resting EMG and end when the EMG amplitude falls to below 2 μV above resting EMG for at least 0.5 seconds.
4. Limb movements within 0.5 seconds preceding the start, or 0.5 following a respiratory event, should not be scored.

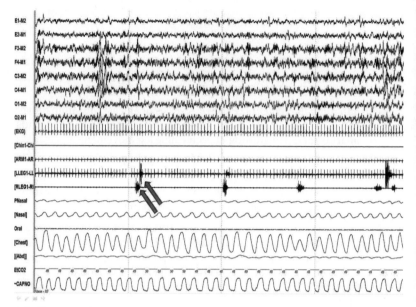

FIGURE 8.27. This 2-minute window demonstrates the same synchronous left and right leg movements in a set of four movements. Two different limbs with movement separated by less than 5 seconds would be considered a single limb movement.

At times, the limb movements are noted to be periodic, but they may not occur at a regular interval. For PLMs, the events must occur in a series and meet the following criteria:

1. A minimum of four consecutive limb movements is necessary to define PLM of sleep.
2. Limb movements must occur for a minimum of 5 seconds, but not longer than 90 seconds between, at the onset of consecutive limb movements.
3. Limb movements of two different limbs separated by less than 5 seconds between movement onsets are counted as a single leg movement.

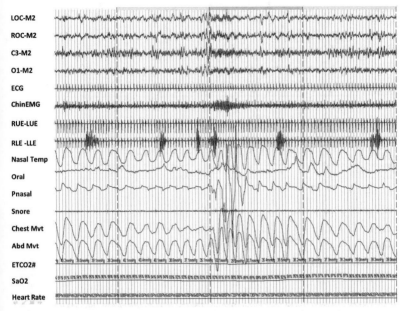

FIGURE 8.28. This is a 2-minute epoch demonstrating PLMS that coexist during hypopneas. The limb movements are noted to occur during the middle of the respiratory event and at the termination of the event. Limb movements near the arousal from the respiratory event are not counted as PLMS.

Periodic leg movements of sleep (PLMS) are recorded during sleep with two EEG cup electrodes placed 2 to 4 cm apart on the anterior tibialis muscle bilaterally. Each leg is recorded in a separate channel. Many periodic movements consist of dorsiflexion of the big toe and foot, but occasionally this can be associated with flexion of the knee and hip. Similar movements can be noted in the arms. These movements are commonly stereotypical and can occur over much of the night. Asynchrony is common and while the majority of limb movements may occur from one leg at a certain time, this pattern may have both time and day variability. The pattern of PLMS is easier to see if a compressed display window is used to include 2 minutes or more.

Leg movements may be associated with arousals or awakenings. Leg movements are scored as being associated with an arousal if they occur within 0.5 seconds of an arousal, regardless of which event occurred initially.

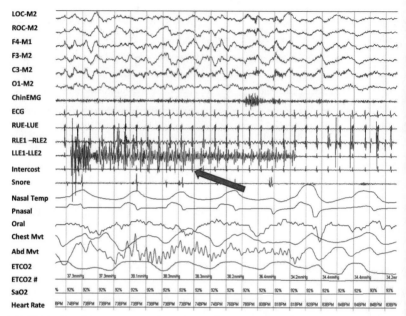

FIGURE 8.29. This is a 30-second epoch demonstrating hypnic foot tremor. Rhythmical EMG artifact is typically seen in one of the lower extremity channels characterized by brief bursts of rhythmical EMG activity. Simultaneous video recording can confirm the tremulous foot movement.

*H*ypnic Foot Tremor is a benign occurrence of rhythmical movement of either foot typically around the onset of sleep. These movements must occur in a train of at least four movements with a frequency range of 0.3 to 4 Hz. Typically, these movements last 250 msec up to a few seconds in duration.

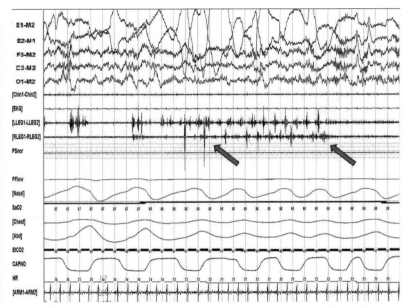

FIGURE 8.30.   This epoch demonstrates ALMA as alternating left and right leg EMG activity (most notable between the arrows). As in this case, the video can demonstrate the limb movements to validate the findings on the PSG.

A related benign movement known as Alternating Leg Muscle Activation (ALMA) reflects foot or leg movement that alternate in a pedaling or ambulatory motion. Similar to most movements, these events must have four movements with a frequency of 0.5 to 3.0Hz during the alternating movements between the legs. Most of these movements last between 100 msec to 3 seconds in duration.

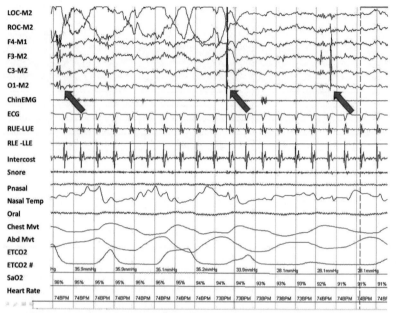

FIGURE 8.31. This 30-second epoch demonstrates myoclonus occurring during REM sleep. This patient had myoclonic jerks in the face and neck throughout Stage R sleep.

Myoclonus is not uncommon during sleep. Characterized by a burst of EMG activity lasting less than 150 msec, myoclonus may be associated with movement involving the large joints of the limbs. For the myoclonus to be identified as abnormal, a minimum of 5 consecutive potentials per minute must be recorded for a minimum of 20 minutes.

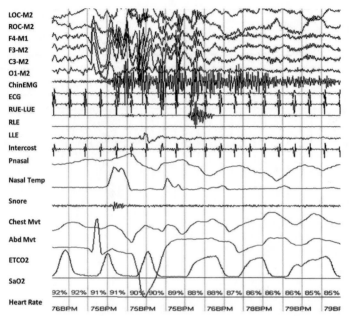

FIGURE 8.32. This 30-second epoch demonstrates phasic bruxism as noted by the rhythmical EMG artifact in the chin and the EEG channels. Simultaneous audio recording revealed typical tooth grinding sounds. Video recording confirmed jaw movements.

Bruxism is brief or sustained teeth clenching identified by an associated increase in chin EMG activity. Most of these events are noted during the transition between wake and sleep. The brief or phasic episodes of bruxism lasts 0.25 to 2 seconds in duration and must have three EMG elevations occur in a regular sequence to be scored. Clenching is evident by tonic elevation of chin EMG activity and is significant when the duration is more than 2 seconds. Many times bruxism is associated with audible click or grinding sound. Additional electrodes placed over the masseter muscle may help identify bruxism.

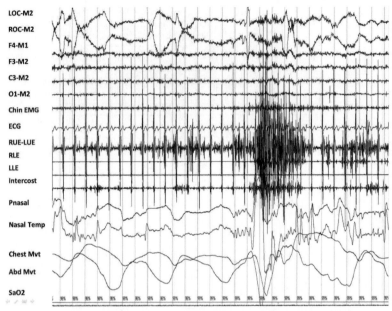

LOC-M2	
ROC-M2	
F4-M1	
F3-M2	
C3-M2	
O1-M2	
Chin EMG	
ECG	
RUE-LUE	
RLE	
LLE	
Intercost	
Pnasal	
Nasal Temp	
Chest Mvt	
Abd Mvt	
SaO2	

FIGURE 8.33. This is a 30-second epoch taken from a PSG of a patient with dream enactment and REM sleep behavior disorder. This segment demonstrates excessive EMG activity in Stage R sleep reflecting an absence of the normal REM sleep atonia. The surge in the EMG activity represents the time that the patient violently swung her arm and verbalized.

REM sleep is associated with skeletal muscle atonia and the absence of atonia may be indicative of a sleep disorder. The presence of muscle tone during Stage R may be sustained or intermittent. Sustained muscle tone (lack of atonia) is scored if at least half of the epoch has increased chin EMG activity above that demonstrated during NREM sleep. Excessive transient muscle activity is determined based upon the presence of muscle activity lasting 0.1 to 5.0 seconds, in at least 5 of the 10 3-second periods of a 30-second epoch. This muscle activity must be at least four times the background muscle activity. The presence of sustained or excessive transient muscle activity is needed to show a loss of atonia in REM sleep. However, there is currently no standard for how many epochs are needed to reach this conclusion. Excessive transient muscle activity may be noted upon video review. Excessive muscle activity in REM sleep may occur with REM suppressing medications (e.g., antidepressants), from alcohol withdrawal, or from a primary sleep disorder such as REM sleep behavior disorder.

A diagnosis of REM sleep behavior disorder requires two features. REM sleep must be evident without atonia on the PSG. In addition, there should be a clinical history or evidence of dream enactment on the PSG. Dream enactment should reflect an obvious behavior that involves movement across large joints and appreciated on video with verbalization noted on audio recording.

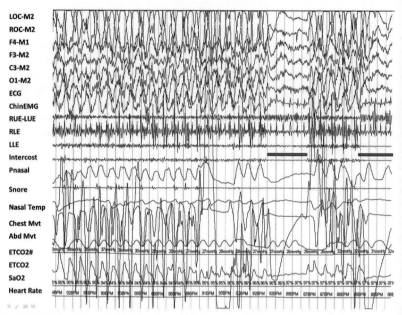

FIGURE 8.34. This epoch demonstrates rhythmical artifact that affects essentially all the EOG, EEG, EMG, and respiratory channels. Of note is that during the interposed brief periods of no artifact (marked by the dark bars), normal background activity is seen.

Rhythmic movement disorder is the presence of metrical stereotypic movement occurring typically in the transition from wake to sleep. These movements may consist of rocking, rolling, headbanging or other rhythmical movements. The movements usually occur in the 0.5 to 2.0 Hz range and a cluster of four successive movements must occur to be scored. These movements are also identifiable by review of the video recording to correlate the source of the rhythmical waveforms in the PSG.

CARDIAC ARRHYTHMIAS

Changes in cardiac function may be encountered during sleep evaluations that include changes in HR or rhythm. Significant apneas or disorders of respiration may produce hypoxia with subsequent measurable changes in the electrocardiogram (EKG). The clinician may subsequently discover subclinical cardiac disturbances that were not previously known for the patient prior to prolonged EKG recording during PSG. Most sleep studies incorporate only one channel of EKG, but cardiac artifact can be seen in multiple channels, including the intercostal and limb EMG as well as the EEG. Cardioballistic movement may also be seen in EEG as well as the respiratory channels.

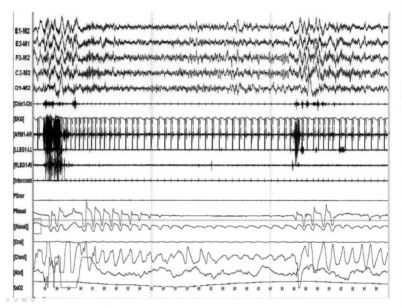

FIGURE 8.35. This 60-second window shows bradycardia on the EKG during an obstructive apnea. This pattern of slowing and rebound tachycardia is common with sleep apnea.

In addition to normal HR and rhythm changes during sleep, potentially serious arrhythmias may be seen. These occur due to fluctuations in the tone of the sympathetic and parasympathetic nervous system during sleep. The most common of these is severe sinus bradycardia. However, atrioventricular block and sinus arrest may also be seen. Hypoxia common with sleep apnea can act as a trigger for cardiac arrhythmias. Cardiac pauses up to 2.5 seconds are considered to have no pathological significance.

Sinus arrhythmia is a frequently observed cardiac dysrhythmia during sleep. It may or may not be associated with respiratory events, but occurs especially in normal young individuals. REM sleep is associated with the wides swings in parasympathetic activity, producing a relative sleep stage-specific increase in sinus pauses. These pauses are considered normal as long as they last under 2.5 seconds and are not associated with cardiac pathology. Periods of asystole lasting 3 seconds should prompt a search for other cardiac abnormalities.

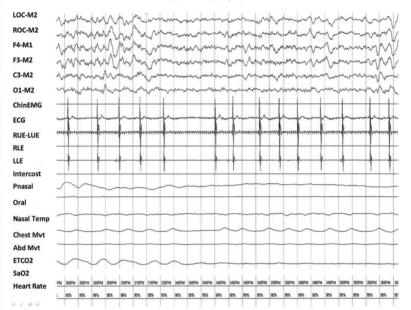

FIGURE 8.36. In contrast to the previous figure, this 30-second epoch demonstrates asystole with a cardiac pause lasting over 3 seconds in NREM sleep. This patient went on to have a cardiac pacemaker placed.

Occasionally, patients will develop potentially malignant arrhythmias such as atrial fibrillation during sleep.

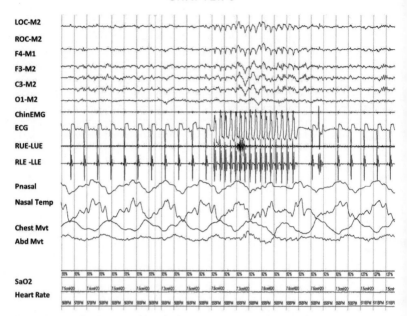

FIGURE 8.37. This 30-second epoch demonstrates a run of ventricular tachycardia in a patient with known ventricular disease. Note the electrocardiac artifact in the EEG channels and the compensatory pause after the run.

Complex arrhythmias are more likely to occur in the early hours, though the reason for this is unclear. Identifying a relationship of the arrhythmia to a respiratory related event may carry clinical implications for the sense of treatment urgency.

EPILEPTIC DISCHARGES

Nocturnal seizures are the predominate manifestation in approximately 20% of patients with epilepsy. Sleep may reveal interictal epileptiform discharges (IEDs) on the EEG portion of the PSG that otherwise were previously unidentified. IEDs are most common in NREM sleep, especially during the transition to Stage N3. REM sleep demonstrates a reduction in the prevalence of IEDs and the field that is involved. As in routine EEG recordings, IEDs must be distinguished pathological spikes from artifact and normal variants. The limited EEG montage and compressed paper speed make identifying these discharges challenging. Expanded EEG montages accenting the frontal and temporal head regions and utilizing a 10-second display window may improve the clinician's ability to recognize these discharges. In addition to the expanded EEG montage and display window, time synchronized high definition infrared camera video and audio recording are helpful in identifying behaviors that may provide information on the semiology of nocturnal events that suggest epilepsy.

(Continued)

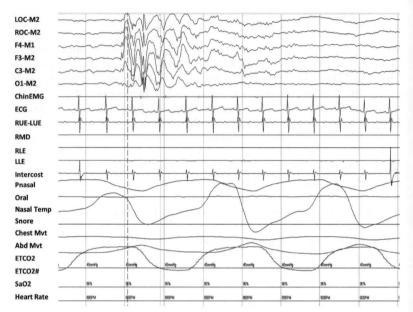

FIGURE 8.38. This is a 10-second epoch demonstrating a generalized spike-and-slow wave discharge in sleep. Note the similarity to a K complex except the presence of a slow wave that distinguishes an IED from a K complex.

(Continued)

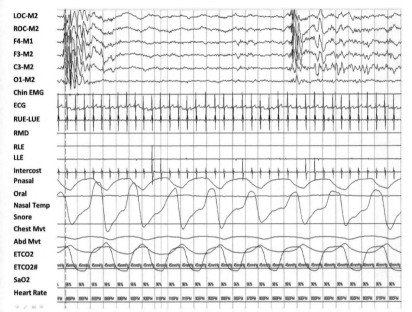

FIGURE 8.39. This is a 30-second epoch demonstrating the same burst of spike-and-slow wave complexes at a normal display speed for a sleep study. Note the additional IEDs in the latter half of the page. This figure illustrates the need to utilize the 10-second display window to identify epileptiform activity.

(Continued)

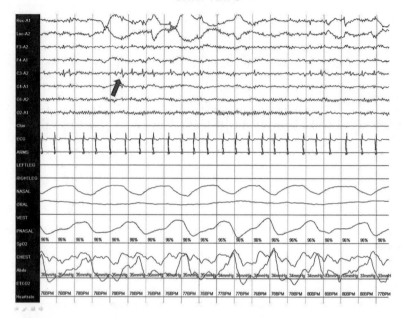

FIGURE 8.40. This figure demonstrates a focal epileptiform discharges emanating from the left hemisphere (arrow) to 10 seconds and increasing the number of electrodes. Note the greater clarity of the IED and its field that is enhanced.

MISCELLANEOUS FINDINGS

Many other patterns can be seen on PSG. Some have diagnostic significance, while others do not. The presence of some findings may suggest additional testing.

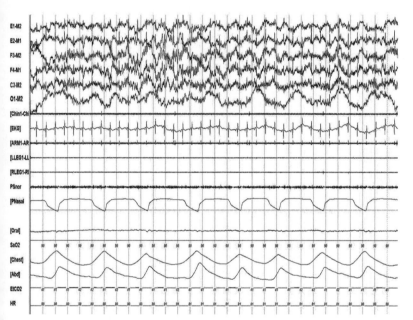

FIGURE 8.41. This 30-second epoch demonstrates an alpha-delta sleep pattern. The alpha frequency activity overrides the delta waves producing a mixture of frequencies. Though the significance of this pattern has been debated, most feel that it has no clear pathological significance.

Alpha-delta sleep pattern is the atypical persistence of an alpha frequency in NREM sleep. The distribution of the alpha activity is more extensive than the normal waking alpha rhythm, and the frequency is usually slower. Underlying sleep spindles, K complexes, and delta waves may be present to confirm the presence of sleep and the stage. Earlier studies noted the occurrence of this pattern in patients with chronic pain syndromes, fibromyalgia, and nonrestorative sleep, but this association and the significance of alpha delta sleep have been questioned since the pattern is found in normal individuals as well.

MULTIPLE SLEEP LATENCY TEST

The multiple sleep latency test (MSLT) is a daytime sleep study in which an individual undergoes a series of five naps scheduled at 2 hour intervals starting 2 hours after the patient first awakens on the day of testing. As a validated test for narcolepsy, this test is an adjunct to overnight polysomnography.

The MSLT is designed to evaluate two features: the time to sleep onset, and the presence of inappropriate REM sleep. The first nap in an MSLT begins 2 hours after the subject awakens from nocturnal sleep. The patient is then placed in bed in a dark room and instructed to allow sleep to come on. If sleep does not occur, the nap trial is ended in 20 minutes. If sleep does occur, the patient is allowed to sleep for 15 minutes. This procedure is repeated at 2-hour intervals throughout the day for a total of five naps.

Sleep onset is scored at the first 30-second epoch of any stage of sleep. For each nap, the sleep-onset latency is determined and if the patient attains Stage R. The mean sleep latency of all the naps is calculated as a total of the sleep latencies that is divided by the total number of naps. If a patient does not attain sleep on a particular nap, the latency is counted as 20 minutes. Also recorded is the number of naps with REM sleep, known as sleep-onset REM periods (SOREM). The diagnosis of narcolepsy is considered if the mean sleep latency is less than 8 minutes and at least two naps demonstrate Stage R sleep.

Maintenance of Wakefulness Test

Similar to the MSLT, the Maintenance of Wakefulness Test (MWT) was developed to estimate ability to remain awake. In this test the subject is in a sitting position in a dimly lit room and instructed to remain awake without stimulating themselves. The subjects must undergo four attempts each, recording for 40 minutes. Once the patient has demonstrated three continuous epochs of Stage N1 sleep or a single epoch of any other stage of sleep, the trial is ended. Although the degree of somnolence and what is acceptable for various activities and occupations is under debate, studies demonstrate that patients are at risk to errors when a mean sleep latency drops below a mean of 8 minutes or less (< 3 standard deviations of the norm). Others consider sleep latencies less than 20 minutes as indicative of sleepiness. Interpretation of these studies must take into account the surrounding information.

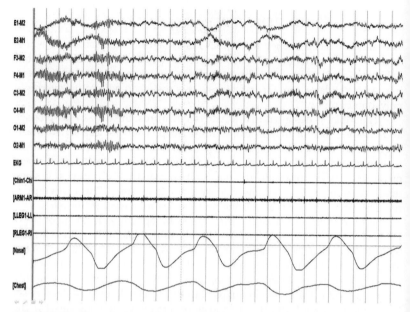

FIGURE 8.42. Upon the loss of the posterior dominant rhythm, stage N1 sleep is seen. In this epoch, note the loss of the alpha background activity and the slow rolling eye movements that are characteristic of stage N1.

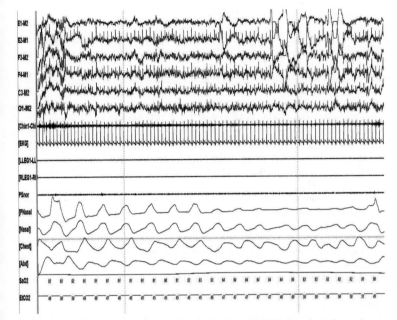

FIGURE 8.43. This 60-second epoch shows the onset of REM sleep from the wake state. Notice the drop in the chin EMG and REMs near the end of this figure.

REM sleep may be present for other reasons than narcolepsy. Subjects who are tested in the nadir of their circadian rhythm, have recently withdrawn from REM suppressing drugs, have been sleep deprived, or have a fever may show REM sleep in this study. SOREM can be frequently seen in individuals who are sleep deprived from sleep apnea. Assurance of at least 6 hours of sleep on PSG the night prior to the MSLT, the absence of another sleep disorder, and review of their sleep schedule and medication list is an important first step prior to performing an MSLT. Patients may also need to have a toxicology screen to evaluate for drugs that may influence the test results.

CHAPTER 8

ADDITIONAL RESOURCES

Aurora RN, Lamm CI, Zak RS, et al. Practice parameters for the non-respiratory indications for polysomnography and multiple sleep latency testing for children. *Sleep*. 2012;35(11):1467-1473.

Aurora RN, Zak RS, Karippot A, et al. Practice parameters for the respiratory indications for polysomnography in children. *Sleep*. 2011;34(3):379-388.

Berry RB, Brooks R, Gamaldo CE, Harding SM, Marcus CL, Vaughn BV for the American Academy of Sleep Medicine. *The AASM Manual for the Scoring of Sleep and Associated Events: Rules, Terminology and Technical Specifications*, Version 2.0. www.aasmnet.org, Darien, Illinois: American Academy of Sleep Medicine; 2012.

Carskadon MA, Dement WC, Mitler MM, Roth T, Westbrook PR, Keenan S. Guidelines for the multiple sleep latency test MSLT): a standard measure of sleepiness. *Sleep*. 1986;9(4):519-524.

Kushida CA, Littner MR, Morgenthaler T, et al. Practice parameters for the indications for polysomnography and related procedures: an update for 2005. *Sleep*. 2005;28(4):499-521.

Littner MR, Kushida C, Wise M, et al. Practice parameters for clinical use of the multiple sleep latency test and the maintenance of wakefulness test. *Sleep*. 2005;28(1):113-121.

Littner MR, Kushida C, Wise M, et al. Practice parameters for clinical use of the multiple sleep latency test and the maintenance of wakefulness test. *Sleep*. 2005;28(1):113-121.

Rechtschaffen A, Kales A, eds. *A Manual of Standardized Terminology, Techniques and Scoring System for Sleep Stages of Human Subjects*. Los Angeles: UCLA Brain Information Service/Brain Research Institute; 1968.

Ruehland WR, Rochford PD, O'Donoghue FJ, Pierce RJ, Singh P, Thornton AT. The new AASM criteria for scoring hypopneas: Impact on the apnea hypopnea index. *Sleep*. 2009;32(2):150-157.

9

Neurophysiologic Intraoperative Monitoring

Aatif M. Husain

Neurophysiologic intraoperative monitoring (NIOM) is increasingly being used to reduce neurologic morbidity during surgeries in which the nervous system is at risk. NIOM allows assessment of neurologic function when the patient cannot be examined. Monitoring waveforms is performed by the neurophysiologist during the active portion of the surgical procedure. Often, the neurophysiologist is able to alert the surgeon of impending injury, allowing the surgeon to modify or reverse the procedure. Several techniques can be used to monitor the nervous system during surgery, and these are chosen depending on the part of the nervous system at risk and type of surgery. Common modalities used for monitoring include brainstem auditory evoked potentials (BAEP), somatosensory evoked potentials (SEP), transcranial electrical motor evoked potentials (MEP), electromyography (EMG), and electroencephalography (EEG). Often, more than one modality will be used; this is known as multimodality monitoring. In this chapter, each modality is shown separately for illustration purposes; in practice, modalities are monitored simultaneously.

BRAINSTEM AUDITORY EVOKED POTENTIALS

BAEP monitoring is used whenever there is potential for injury to the vestibulocochlear nerve or its pathways. Common procedures during which BAEP monitoring is used include microvascular decompression (MVD) surgery for trigeminal neuralgia and hemifacial spasm and cerebellopontine angle (CPA) tumor surgery. It may also be used during other types of brainstem surgery. BAEP monitoring has been shown to reduce the incidence of hearing loss associated with MVD surgeries.

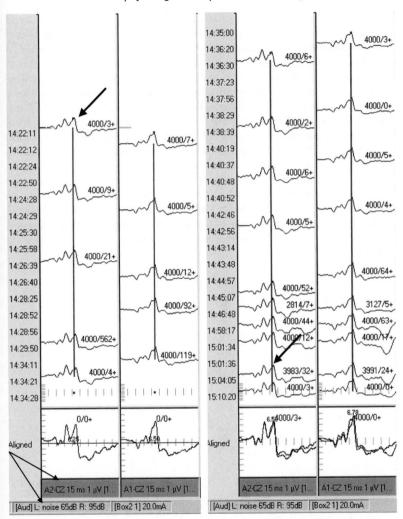

FIGURE 9.1. This is intraoperative brainstem auditory evoked potentials (BAEP) monitoring data that showed no significant change in waveforms throughout the surgery.

(Continued)

During surgery the BAEP ipsilateral to the side of surgery is monitored closely. Changes in the latencies and amplitudes of the wave I and wave V in relation to the baseline are noted. The contralateral median nerve SEP is also periodically monitored. This evaluates conduction in the dorsal column pathways in the brainstem which lie close to the vestibulocochlear pathway. This type of multimodality monitoring is particularly useful in CPA tumor surgery. At times, the contralateral BAEP and ipsilateral median SEP are also checked for comparison purposes. The example (Figure 9.1) is from a 63-year-old patient undergoing MVD surgery for right-sided trigeminal neuralgia. BAEPs from right ear stimulation are shown. Stimulation parameters are noted at the bottom of the graph as is the montage (thin arrows). Notice that the latency and amplitude of the wave V did not change significantly during the procedure (thick arrows). The vertical line is drawn on the wave V; notice the consistency with which the wave V falls on this line, indicating no significant change in latency. This monitoring did not suggest permanent damage to the vestibulocochlear pathway ipsilateral to the side of surgery.

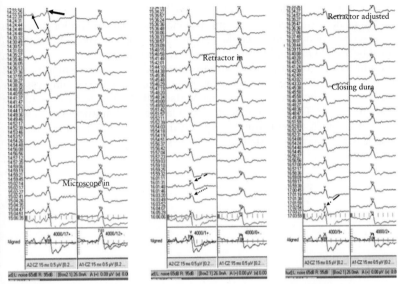

FIGURE 9.2. This is intraoperative brainstem auditory evoked potentials (BAEP) monitoring data showing a small increase in wave V latency and a 50% decrease in amplitude.

During BAEP monitoring, a wave V latency prolongation of 1 msec or an amplitude decrement of 50% is considered significant (latency shift is considered more important). Three possible mechanisms can account for a change in the BAEP. First, one must consider technical issues, then global physiological changes such as anesthesia or blood pressure variation, and finally surgically induced change. The pattern of change of the BAEP (i.e., which waves are affected) helps determine the etiology. If the change is thought to be surgery, induced, the surgeon must be alerted immediately. During MVD surgery, the cerebellum is retracted to expose the CPA. This causes stretch injury to the vestibulocochlear nerve, which if severe enough can lead to hearing loss. BAEP are commonly performed in MVD to prevent this complication. In the sample above, the patient is undergoing MVD for right trigeminal neuralgia. At the start of the case, waves I (thin arrow) and V (thick arrow) are clearly identified. Soon after placement of the cerebellar retractor, there is prolongation of the wave V latency (notice the dot placed on the peak of wave V at baseline). The maximum latency prolongation is 0.6 msec, which does not reach the critical 1 msec point at which the surgeon must be alerted (dashed arrow). However, there is a significant decrease in the amplitude (greater than 50%) (dotted arrow). The surgeon is alerted, and he repositions the cerebellar retractor. After completing the decompression, the retractor is removed and the wave V gradually returns to baseline (dash and dot arrow). There is change in wave I latency and morphology as well, but not as much as with wave V. The return of the BAEP to near baseline suggests that permanent damage to the vestibulocochlear pathway ipsilateral to the side of surgery did not occur.

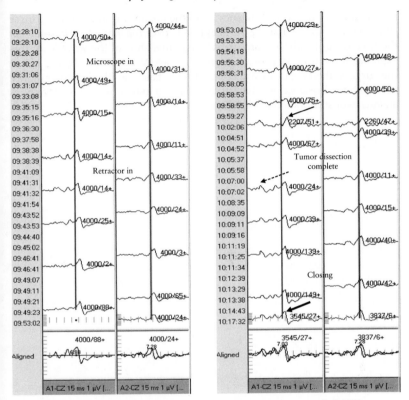

FIGURE 9.3. This is intraoperative brainstem auditory evoked potentials (BAEP) monitoring data showing a wave V latency prolongation of 1.5 msec and amplitude reduction of more than 50%.

A 1.0 msec prolongation of wave V latency is considered significant, and the surgeon should be alerted. A persistent 1.0 msec or worsening latency shift is more likely to be associated with postoperative hearing loss. More recent data suggests that latency shifts should be interpreted based on the underlying disease state. For example, in patients with CPA tumors, even smaller latency shifts may be clinically significant. In this sample from a patient undergoing resection of a left acoustic neuroma, there is gradual prolongation of the wave V latency, with the maximum shift being 1.5 msec (thin arrow). Notice that the vertical line is over the wave V at baseline; at the time of tumor dissection, there is maximal shift of the wave V. In this example, there is no significant change in wave V amplitude. By the end of the surgery, the latency of wave V is close to baseline (thick arrow) (notice vertical line). Presence of wave I at the time of maximal wave V shift implies adequacy of stimulation (dashed arrow).

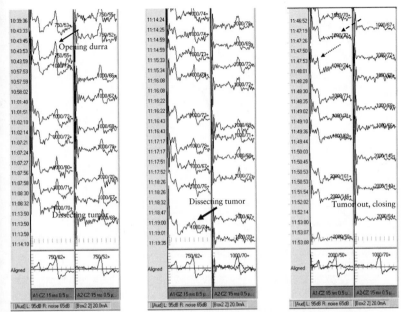

FIGURE 9.4. This is intraoperative brainstem auditory evoked potentials (BAEP) monitoring data showing loss of wave V during cerebellopontine angle (CPA) tumor dissection without return by the end of the surgery.

Loss of the wave V waveform is the most severe type of change that can occur with intraoperative BAEP monitoring. If it does not return by the end of the surgery, the patient is likely to have postoperative hearing loss. However, loss of the wave V is not incompatible with preserved hearing (i.e., false-positive). When complete loss of wave V occurs suddenly, it is usually due to interruption of vascular supply of the vestibulocochlear nerve. If the loss is gradual, the etiology is more likely to be either mechanical or thermal trauma to the nerve. In the above sample of BAEP monitoring during left acoustic neuroma surgery, there is a robust wave V at the start of the case (thin arrow). However as tumor dissection progresses, there is gradual loss of amplitude (thick arrow) and eventually there is complete loss of the wave V (dashed arrow). It does not return by the end of the case. The preserved wave I (dotted arrow) confirms that this change is not due to technical reasons.

305

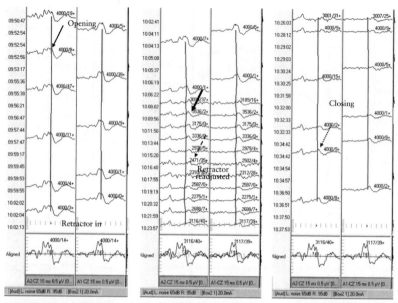

FIGURE 9.5. This is intraoperative brainstem auditory evoked potentials (BAEP) monitoring data showing loss of wave V during microvascular decompression (MVD) with return by the end of the surgery.

Loss of wave V followed by recovery before the end of the surgery suggests that hearing will be preserved. This is especially true in patients undergoing MVD surgery. In the sample above, the patient is undergoing a MVD for right trigeminal neuralgia. A wave V is noted at baseline (thin arrow), however, with cerebellar retraction there is gradual latency prolongation up to 0.7 msec and amplitude loss (thick arrow) and finally disappearance (dashed arrow). Once the retractor is removed, there is gradual recovery of the wave V (dotted arrow).

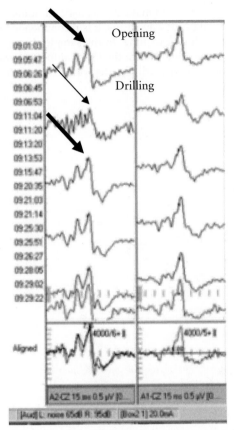

FIGURE 9.6. This is intraoperative brainstem auditory evoked potentials (BAEP) monitoring data showing loss of wave V during drilling of bone.

As noted previously, with surgery induced changes, BAEP changes can occur due to technical issues and overall physiological changes. One such technical issue arises with bone drilling during exposure. The drill makes a loud noise which can mask the acoustic stimulus of the BAEP. This may cause loss of the BAEP waveforms. It is recommended that BAEP averaging be suspended during drilling. In the sample above, BAEP averaging is continued during drilling. Notice the lower amplitude wave V waveform (thin arrow). Before and after drilling, the wave V waveform is robust (thick arrows).

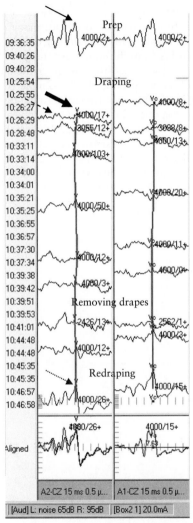

FIGURE 9.7. This is intraoperative brainstem auditory evoked potentials (BAEP) monitoring data showing loss of wave V soon after draping the patient.

(Continued)

Many technical problems can lead to loss of BAEP waveforms. Inadequacy of stimulation may occur for many different reasons. A relatively common cause is kinking or clamping of the tubing used to transmit the acoustic stimulus from the sound generator to the ear. Obstruction of this tubing prevents the clicks from reaching the auditory system, and consequently a BAEP is not produced. The sample (Figure 9.7) is from a patient undergoing MVD for right trigeminal neuralgia. Soon after positioning, the baseline response was obtained and revealed a robust wave V waveform (thin arrow). However, soon after draping the patient, there was sudden loss of the wave V (thick arrow). Notice also that the wave I also disappeared (dashed arrow). The absence of all BAEP waveforms suggested inadequacy of stimulation. After the clamps of the drape were removed, the BAEP response returned (dotted arrow).

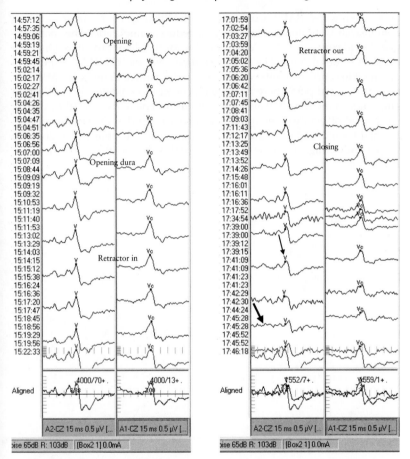

FIGURE 9.8. This is intraoperative brainstem auditory evoked potentials (BAEP) monitoring data showing latency prolongation and amplitude decrement of the wave V toward the end of the surgery.

The auditory stimulator which is secured in the external auditory canal can be inadvertently pulled out, especially towards the end of a long surgery. With dislodgement of the stimulator, lower stimulation intensity is provoking the BAEP. Consequently, BAEP may be misinterpreted as demonstrating prolonged latency and reduced amplitude. The technologist should confirm that the change is due to stimulator problems. Once the problem is found, it must be corrected; if possible another BAEP response is obtained to confirm no interval change. In this patient undergoing MVD for right trigeminal pain, there is gradual prolongation of latency and drop in amplitude of the wave V waveform towards the end of the case (thin arrow). At the end of the case, the technologist confirmed that the stimulator tubing had been dislodged. Notice that as the wave V disappears, so does the wave I, indicating a peripheral etiology for this change (thick arrow).

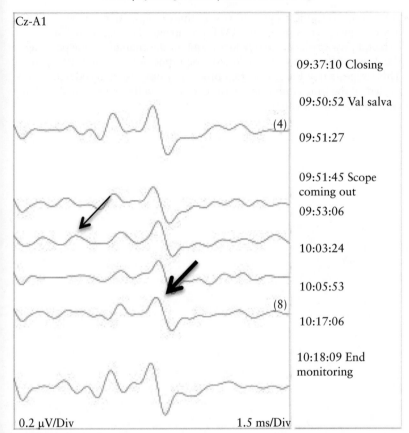

Cz-A1

09:37:10 Closing

09:50:52 Val salva

(4)   09:51:27

09:51:45 Scope coming out

09:53:06

10:03:24

10:05:53

(8)   10:17:06

10:18:09 End monitoring

0.2 μV/Div   1.5 ms/Div

FIGURE 9.9. This is intraoperative monitoring data obtained from stimulation of the left ear. The surgery being performed was microvascular decompression for trigeminal neuralgia for the right ear. Notice the drop in amplitude of the wave V of the brainstem auditory evoked potentials (BAEP) obtained after stimulation of the left ear (thick arrow). The BAEP from the operative side (right) was unchanged.

As noted above, technical issues must be considered when changes in BAEP are noted. When right sided microvascular decompression is being performed, it would be very unlikely for the left-sided BAEP to change at the time of closing, as was the case in this example (thick arrow). Without any changes in the right-sided BAEP, physiological changes, such as a drop in blood pressure, are unlikely to account for the change. A clue pointing to the cause of the change is the loss of amplitude of the wave I (thin arrow). This suggests that the stimulation probe may have been dislodged. As suspected, at the time of undraping, the ear insert on the left side had partially come out of the ear canal.

SOMATOSENSORY EVOKED POTENTIALS

SEP monitoring is most often used for monitoring the spinal cord during surgeries in which it may be at risk. In scoliosis surgery, SEP has been shown to reduce neurologic morbidity. SEP can also be used during surgeries on the spinal cord, brainstem, and thoracic aorta. Additionally, median SEP have been used for cortical localization (discussed later). Tibial SEP are used when surgery involves risk to the spinal cord below the lower cervical level. In such cases, median or ulnar SEP can be used as a control. For surgeries involving risk to the upper to mid cervical spinal cord, median or ulnar SEP are used (ulnar preferentially used if C6-7 region is at risk). Subcortical (P14/N18 for upper, P31/N34 for lower) and cortical (N20 for upper, P37 for lower) waveforms are followed during surgery.

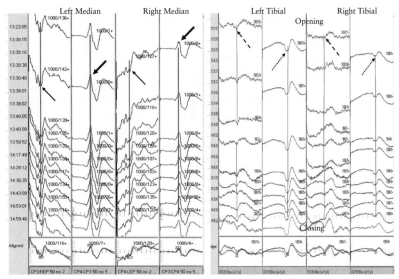

FIGURE 9.10. This is intraoperative median and tibial somatosensory evoked potentials (SEP) monitoring data showing no significant change during the procedure.

As with BAEP, SEP changes can be induced by technical problems, general physiological changes, and surgery induced damage. The pattern of change helps localize the problem. It should be remembered that SEP monitors the dorsal column pathway (posterior aspect of spinal cord) and serves only as a surrogate marker for the corticospinal pathways. In many instances, SEP monitoring is done in conjunction with other types of monitoring. In the sample shown here, the patient is undergoing posterior spinal fusion for scoliosis. The median SEP are being used as a control. Both subcortical (P14, thin arrows) (first and third columns) and cortical (N20, thick arrows) (second and fourth columns) responses are displayed. Tibial SEP are followed closely. Subcortical (P31, dashed arrows) (first and third columns) and cortical (P37, dotted arrows) (second and fourth columns) are displayed. No significant change in the responses is noted, and neurologic morbidity is not anticipated.

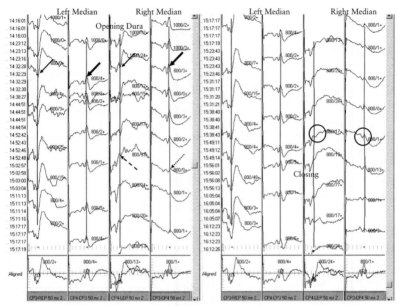

FIGURE 9.11. This is intraoperative median somatosensory evoked potentials (SEP) monitoring data showing gradual loss of the subcortical and cortical waveforms after right sided stimulation.

A significant change in SEP is 50% decrease in amplitude or a 10% increase in latency. Unlike BAEP, with SEP an amplitude change is more significant. When such a change occurs, and technical and general physiological causes have been excluded, the surgeon should be alerted. The sample above is from a patient undergoing upper cervical syringomelia decompression. Median subcortical (first and third columns) and cortical (second and fourth columns) responses are displayed. At the start of the case, robust subcortical (thin arrows) and cortical (thick arrows) responses are seen. As the surgery progresses, there is gradual loss of amplitude of the subcortical (dashed arrow) and cortical (dotted arrow) waveforms obtained after right-sided stimulation. At the end of surgery these responses are almost completely lost (circles). This patient is likely to have postoperative dysfunction of the dorsal column pathway of the right median nerve.

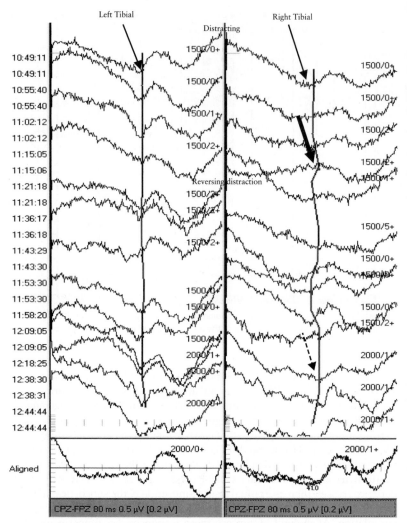

FIGURE 9.12. This is intraoperative tibial somatosensory evoked potentials (SEP) monitoring data showing transient loss of the cortical waveform after right tibial nerve stimulation.

(*Continued*)

During scoliosis surgery implantation of hardware (sublaminar wires and hooks) and distraction can lead to spinal cord injury. Monitoring SEP allows determination of when such compromise is imminent. The sample shown above is from a patient undergoing a posterior spinal fusion for scoliosis. Cortical (P37) waveforms (thin arrows) are seen at the start of distraction. However, soon thereafter the cortical response obtained after stimulation of the right tibial nerve has a decrease in amplitude and is difficult to identify (thick arrow); the surgeon is alerted. After the surgeon reverses the distraction, the responses improve (dashed arrow). Without SEP monitoring, the surgeon would not have been aware of the spinal cord compromise, possibly leading to neurologic morbidity.

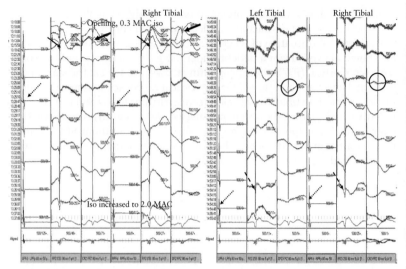

FIGURE 9.13. This is intraoperative tibial somatosensory evoked potentials (SEP) monitoring data showing gradual loss of the cortical waveforms with use of halogenated anesthetics.

There are many systemic factors that can affect SEP. One of the most common such factors is anesthetics. Cortical waveforms, particularly of the tibial SEP, are very sensitive to inhalational (halogenated agents and nitrous oxide) anesthetics. Often, concentrations of 1.0 minimum alveolar concentration (MAC) can eliminate the cortical responses. Subcortical responses are more resilient to inhalational anesthetics and often can be followed in cases in which such anesthetics are used. The patient shown here is undergoing posterior spinal fusion for scoliosis. At the start of the case, isoflurane 0.3 MAC is used. Well defined subcortical (thin arrows) and cortical (thick arrows) responses are seen. However, when the isoflurane is increased to 2.0 MAC, there is obliteration of the cortical response bilaterally (circles). Notice that the subcortical responses persist despite the increase in anesthetics (dashed arrows). The first and fourth column is the popliteal fossa (PF) response (dotted arrows) which indicates adequacy of stimulation.

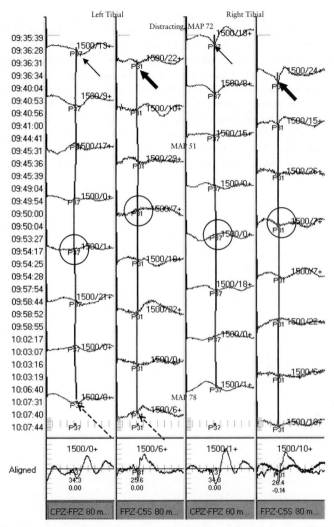

FIGURE 9.14. This is intraoperative tibial somatosensory evoked potentials (SEP) monitoring data showing intermittent loss of cortical and subcortical waveforms with fluctuating blood pressure.

(Continued)

A drop in blood pressure can affect SEP waveforms, causing a decrease in amplitude of the cortical and subcortical potentials. This is likely due to hypoperfusion of the spinal cord. The sample (Figure 9.14) is from a patient undergoing posterior spinal fusion for scoliosis. The first and third columns display the cortical (P37) waveforms while the second and fourth columns display the subcortical (P31/N34) waveforms. When the mean arterial pressure (MAP) is about 70, both cortical (thin arrows) and subcortical (thick arrows) waveforms are seen. However, when the pressure drops to about 50, there is significant amplitude reduction of the waveforms (circles). When the pressure is raised, the responses return (dashed arrows). In this patient, monitoring helped keep the MAP somewhat higher than would have been chosen otherwise.

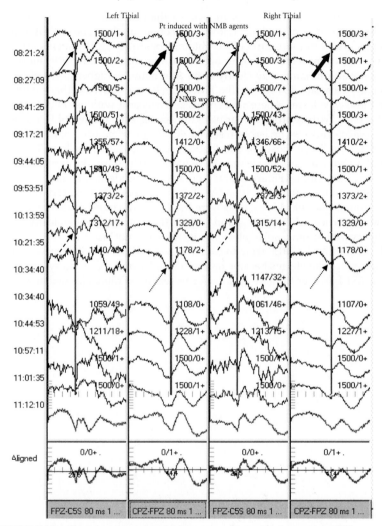

FIGURE 9.15. This is intraoperative tibial somatosensory evoked potentials (SEP) monitoring data showing poor reproducibility of the subcortical waveforms and preserved cortical waveforms with wearing off of neuromuscular blocking agents.

(Continued)

Subcortical SEP waveforms are smaller than cortical ones and harder to resolve with averaging. With EMG contamination, subcortical waveforms are even more difficult to obtain. Consequently, if patients are not given neuromuscular blocking agents during surgery, often the subcortical waveforms cannot be clearly seen. Alternatively, higher doses of anesthetic gases can also reduce the EMG activity and increase the resolution of these waveforms. There are benefits and concerns with use of both types of agents. With neuromuscular blocking agents, even though SEP subcortical waveforms can be easily resolved, MEP cannot be used. On the other hand, with higher doses of anesthetic gases, though there is less EMG, the SEP waveforms' amplitude may be reduced, particularly the cortical waveforms. The sample (Figure 9.15) is from a patient undergoing anterior cervical decompression and fixation (ACDF) for stenosis. At the start of the case, neuromuscular blocking agents were used for intubation. At this time both the subcortical (thin arrows) and cortical (thick arrows) were clearly seen. However, neuromuscular blocking agents were not used for the remainder of the case as MEP were to be used. As the EMG activity returned, the subcortical waveforms became harder to resolve and more "noisy" (dashed arrows), however the cortical waveforms remained robust (dotted arrows).

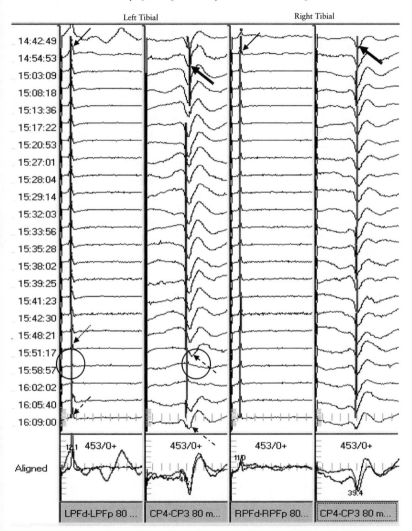

FIGURE 9.16. This is intraoperative tibial somatosensory evoked potentials (SEP) monitoring data showing loss of popliteal fossa (PF) and P37 waveforms after left sided stimulation.

(Continued)

In addition to surgical and physiological factors, technical issues must be considered whenever there is a change in waveforms. Whereas physiological changes, such as anesthetic and blood pressure changes, are more likely to affect all SEP responses, technical issues are more likely to produce more focal changes. The example (Figure 9.16) is from a patient undergoing a thoracic laminectomy for removal of an extradural spinal lesion. The first and third column show the PF (peripheral) response, whereas the second and fourth column show the P37 (cortical) response. Initially robust, PF (thin arrows) and P37 (thick arrows) responses are seen bilaterally. At 15:51:17 mild latency prolongation of the P37 after left tibial nerve stimulation is noted (dashed arrow). Notice also that the ipsilateral PF response amplitude is reduced (dotted arrow). Soon, thereafter, both the PF and P37 responses disappear (circles). Loss of the PF response suggests a problem with adequate stimulation on the left side. The technologist checked the stimulating needles and found that they had been dislodged. Readjusting the stimulating needles resulted in return of both the PF and P37 responses (dashed-dotted arrows).

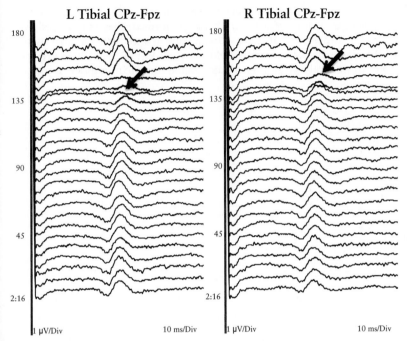

FIGURE 9.17. This is tibial somatosensory evoked potentials (SEP) intraoperative monitoring data in a 16-year-old undergoing posterior spinal fusion for scoliosis. The waveforms at the bottom of the page were acquired earlier, and the graphs on the top of the screen were acquired later. Notice the transient loss of cortical waveforms (thick arrows).

In the above patient, cortical P37 waveforms are being displayed. Loss of cortical waveforms during scoliosis surgery, especially during spinal column manipulation, may be due to traumatic injury to the spinal cord. When this occurs, subcortical waveforms decrease in amplitude as well. Cortical waveforms may decrease in amplitude with a change in anesthetics as well, such as if inhalational anesthetics are started or increased. This will result in little change in the subcortical waveforms. Thus, subcortical waveforms can be used to help differentiate between these two possible mechanisms of waveform change. If MEP are being performed, they may also show a change. However, the latter may change due to anesthetic regimen change. In this case, the subcortical waveforms were lost as well. Whenever possible, subcortical waveforms should be monitored in addition to cortical waveforms.

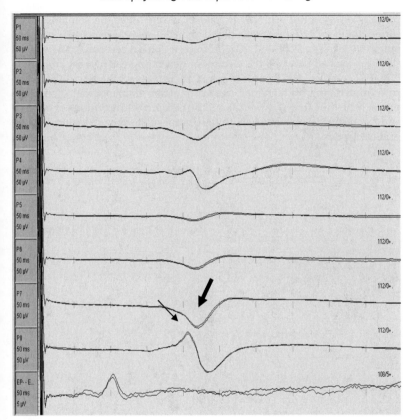

FIGURE 9.18. This is an intraoperative median somatosensory evoked potentials (SEP) used to localize the central sulcus.

SEP has been used to localize the central sulcus in patients undergoing neurosurgery near the motor strip or for patients undergoing stimulator implantations for facial pain. For recording these potentials, a grid with at least 8 contacts is placed on the exposed cortex. The contralateral median nerve is stimulated and recordings made sequentially from the various contacts on the grid. An N20 waveform is seen over the somatosensory cortex while a P22 (sometimes called the P20) waveform is seen over the motor cortex. The N20 and P22 produce a "phase reversal." The central sulcus is located between the electrodes generating the highest amplitude N20/P22 complex. The sample (Figure 9.18) is from a patient with left facial pain undergoing intracranial neurostimulator implantation. There are robust N20 (thin arrow) as well as a P22 (thick arrow) waveforms at points 8 and 7 of the grid, respectively with the central sulcus lying between the two grid electrodes.

MOTOR EVOKED POTENTIALS

MEP are obtained by electrically stimulating the brain through the scalp and recording the response over the spinal cord (direct, D, and indirect, I, waves), nerves (nerve MEP), or muscles (muscle MEP). The impulse travels in the corticospinal tract and is a much better predictor of paraparesis than SEP. Most often recordings are made from small hand and foot muscles. Spinal recordings (for D and I waves) are used less often due to their invasive nature. When recording MEP from muscles, a train of high voltage (200–600 V) stimuli is applied to the scalp. The train summates at the anterior horn cell level and produces a muscle MEP. Large series have demonstrated the safety of MEP. MEP are a useful adjunct to SEP monitoring, and with both modalities, both the anterior and posterior aspects of the spinal cord can be monitored. Inhalational anesthetics suppress the anterior horn cells, and consequently their use makes obtaining MEP more difficult. Intravenous anesthetics (propofol and opiods) are preferred when MEP monitoring is to be used.

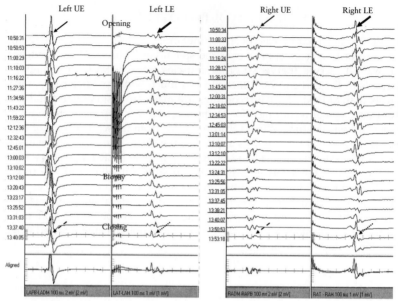

FIGURE 9.19. This is intraoperative motor evoked potentials (MEP) monitoring data showing stable responses in the upper and lower extremities.

The above sample is from a patient undergoing biopsy of a cervical lesion. Robust MEP responses are obtained from both upper (thin arrows) and lower (thick arrows) extremities at the start of the case. Towards the end of the case, similarly robust upper (dashed arrows) and lower (dotted arrows) extremity responses are noted.

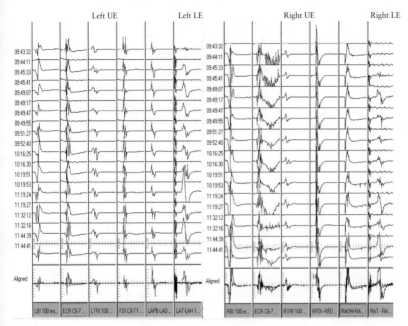

FIGURE 9.20. This is intraoperative motor evoked potentials (MEP) monitoring data showing stable responses in several upper and a single lower extremity muscle.

During surgeries in which the spinal cord is at risk, monitoring one upper and one or two lower extremity muscles is sufficient. However, in patients in whom nerve roots as well as the spinal cord is at risk (e.g., cervical stenosis/myelopathy), monitoring multiple muscles with varying root innervation may be helpful. This can allow detection of not only spinal cord injury, but also injury to individual nerve roots. In the sample above, the biceps brachii (first column), extensor carpi radialis longus (second column), triceps (third column), first dorsal interosseous (fourth column), abductor pollicis brevis (fifth column), and anterior tibialis/abductor hallucis (sixth column) muscles are monitored in a patient undergoing multilevel cervical decompression. Robust responses are noted throughout the case, suggesting no radicular or spinal cord compromise. Notice that responses are present in alternate traces. This is because MEP stimulation can be applied selectively to one hemisphere, producing a response only on the contralateral side.

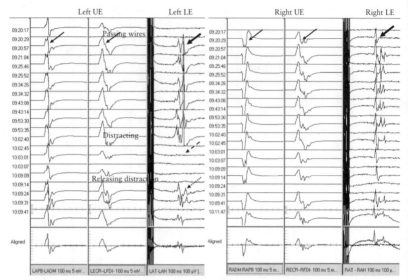

FIGURE 9.21. This is intraoperative motor evoked potentials (MEP) monitoring data showing stable responses in both upper extremities and the right lower extremity, but there is transient loss of the MEP response in the left lower extremity.

Unlike BAEP and SEP, there is disagreement as to what constitutes a significant MEP change. Some investigators suggest that if the stimulation intensity has to be increased during the case to elicit the same response, that is a significant change. Others suggest that unless the response is completely lost, regardless of the stimulation intensity, the change is not significant. In the author's practice, a significant response is one in which the response disappears completely or by at least 80%. The patient shown above was undergoing posterior spinal fusion for scoliosis. At the start of the case MEP responses are noted in both upper (first two columns of each graph, thin arrows) and lower (last column in each graph, thick arrows) extremities. With distraction there was loss of the left lower extremity MEP (dashed arrow). The surgeon was notified and the distraction was relaxed. The MEP returned (dotted arrow).

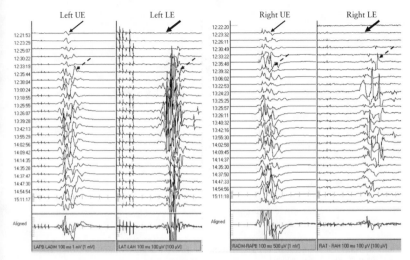

FIGURE 9.22. This is intraoperative motor evoked potentials (MEP) monitoring data showing absent MEP responses in the lower extremities initially; however, later in the case MEP to all four extremities were stable.

MEP are very sensitive to inhalational anesthetics and neuromuscular blocking agents. Especially if these drugs are given in boluses, as when inducing a patient, the affect on MEP is remarkable. Low doses of both, if consistently maintained, may be compatible with successful MEP monitoring. However, in this situation reliability of the MEP monitoring is decreased. The above patient was undergoing spinal cord tumor biopsy. He was induced with neuromuscular blocking agents. Initially, upper extremity MEP (first column) were seen (thin arrows), but lower extremity responses were absent (thick arrows). Since further boluses of neuromuscular blocking agents were not administered, after a few minutes robust MEP were seen for both upper and lower extremities (dashed arrows). Notice also that the morphology of the MEP responses in a given limb changes. This is a normal finding.

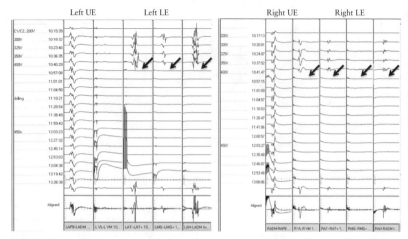

FIGURE 9.23. This is motor evoked potentials (MEP) monitoring data showing sudden loss of MEP responses in both lower extremities (arrows).

This patient was undergoing excision of tumor around the thoracic aorta. As the surgeon was dissecting tumor, a strand of tissue that was thought to be a tumor was cut, but was instead ultimately suspected to involve a vascular supply to the thoracic spinal cord. There was sudden loss of MEP in both lower extremities. MEP in the upper extremities remained stable. As noted previously, there can be many reasons for changes in MEP. The lack of any change in upper extremity MEP and total loss of lower extremity MEP, however, implies injury to the spinal cord. The acute nature of this change suggests that the injury was vascular. It would be very unusual for physiologic changes, such as blood pressure change, or anesthetics to affect the lower extremity MEP so dramatically and not cause any change in the upper extremity MEP. Tibial SEP are also expected to change when this happens (as they did in this case), but that change typically will lag behind the change in MEP in the case of vascular injury to the spinal cord. The patient awoke with a neurological deficit involving weakness of both lower extremities.

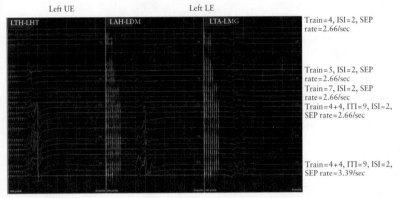

Left UE Left LE

Train=4, ISI=2, SEP rate=2.66/sec

Train=5, ISI=2, SEP rate=2.66/sec
Train=7, ISI=2, SEP rate=2.66/sec
Train=4+4, ITI=9, ISI=2, SEP rate=2.66/sec

Train=4+4, ITI=9, ISI=2, SEP rate=3.39/sec

FIGURE 9.24. This is motor evoked potentials (MEP) monitoring data showing an increase in the amplitude of the MEP responses in the upper and lower extremities when double train stimulation was used.

MEP can be difficult to obtain in some patients with myelopathy and in young children. In these situations, MEP stimulation can be modified to increase the chances of getting MEP that can be monitored during the surgery. This can be done by partially depolarizing the anterior horn cells before the MEP stimulus arrives; this is called facilitation. This allows easier depolarization of the anterior horn cells, enhancing the ability to elicit a muscle MEP. One way this can be done is to use double train stimulation. With double train stimulation, the first train of four impulses serves to partially depolarize the anterior horn cells, and the second train depolarizes them completely, eliciting the muscle MEP. In the example above, note that when a train of seven stimuli are administered, a left upper extremity response is seen (purple), but the responses in the lower extremity are very small and not reliable. Thereafter, a double train of 4 + 4 stimuli is delivered, and much more robust upper and lower extremity responses are noted (especially in the left foot – middle column). The inter-train interval (ITI) must be timed appropriately. If it is too short, the second train will fall on the refractory period of the anterior horn cells. If it is too late, the partial depolarizing effects of the first train will disappear. An ITI of eight to ten is recommended.

ELECTROMYOGRAPHY

Monitoring of the peripheral nervous system can be performed with free running EMG, stimulated EMG, or nerve action potentials. To record free running (or stimulated) EMG, needle or wire electrodes are placed in muscles innervated by nerves that are at risk. Significant injury to nerves during dissection produces high frequency discharges called neurotonic discharges. Short bursts of neurotonic discharges signify transient nerve irritation; if persistent, the injury may be irreversible.

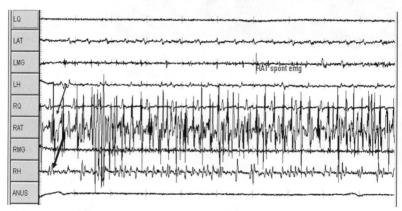

FIGURE 9.25. This is intraoperative free running EMG monitoring data showing a neurotonic discharge arising from the right anterior tibialis muscle.

This example is from a patient undergoing tethered cord release surgery. The channels are monitoring left vastus lateralis, left anterior tibialis, left medial gastrocnemius, left semitendinosis, right vastus lateralis, right anterior tibialis, right medial gastrocnemius, right semitendinosis, and anus muscles with needle electrodes. One second is displayed. There is a high frequency run of discharges consistent with a neurotonic discharge arising from the right anterior tibialis muscle (thin arrow) and to a lesser extent from the right hamstring muscle (thick arrow). Upon hearing the discharge, the surgeon stopped dissecting and irrigated the surgical field; the neurotonic discharge stopped.

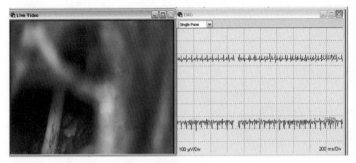

FIGURE 9.26.   This is intraoperative free running EMG activity displaying on-going neurotonic discharges in the facial nerve channels (orbicularis oculi and oris).

Ongoing neurotonic discharges can indicate injury to the nerve. These have also been referred to as type A trains. The longer the discharge, the worse the injury is likely to be involving the facial nerve. Pausing during dissection and irrigating the surgical field may reduce the frequency of these discharges. On the left is an intraoperative photograph of the facial nerve that was potentially being injured during this case.

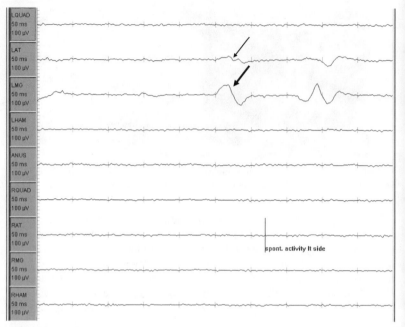

FIGURE 9.27. This is intraoperative free running EMG monitoring data showing occasional spontaneous muscle activity arising from the left anterior tibialis and medial gastrocnemius muscles.

Minor irritation of a nerve often causes spontaneous firing of motor units supplied by that nerve. While monitoring free running EMG, an abnormality is manifested by low frequency, short discharges. These discharges are not associated with postoperative morbidity. The above sample is displaying 100 msec of data from a patient undergoing tethered cord release surgery. The left vastus lateralis, left anterior tibialis, left medial gastrocnemius, left semitendinosis, anus, right vastus lateralis, right anterior tibialis, right medial gastrocnemius, and right semitendinosis muscles are being monitored. During irrigation, low frequency discharges are noted in the left anterior tibialis (thin arrow) and medial gastrocnemius (thick arrow) muscles. They disappeared after a few seconds.

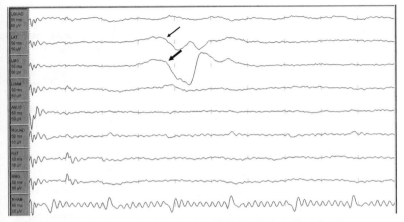

FIGURE 9.28. This is intraoperative stimulated EMG monitoring data showing a response in the left anterior tibialis and medial gastrocnemius muscles.

Stimulated EMG can be used to identify neural structures during surgery. For example, if a tumor is surrounding neural tissue, focal stimulation in various areas of the tumor can be helpful in determining where neural elements are present. Alternatively, often when anatomy is not clear, structures in the surgical field can be stimulated and, according to the pattern of response seen, they can be correctly identified. In the example above, stimulation of a nerve root produced a triggered response in the left anterior tibialis (thin arrow) and the medial gastrocnemius (thick arrow) muscles. The most likely root stimulated is the left L5. This is a 100 msec sample, and the montage is left vastus lateralis, left anterior tibialis, left medial gastrocnemius, left semitendinosis, anus, right vastus lateralis, right anterior tibialis, right medial gastrocnemius, and right semitendinosis muscles.

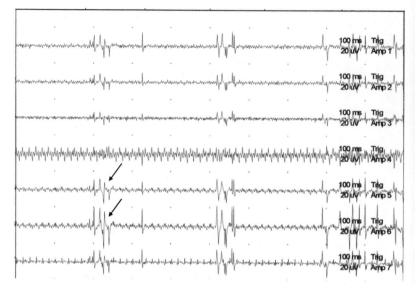

FIGURE 9.29. This is intraoperative EMG monitoring data showing an artifact that resembles a neurotonic discharge.

As with other types of monitoring, artifacts are common in EMG monitoring as well. Differentiating artifacts from neurotonic discharges is very important. The above sample is from a patient undergoing tethered cord release surgery. One second is displayed. The montage is left anterior tibialis, left medial gastrocnemius, left semitendinosis, anus, right anterior tibialis, right medial gastrocnemius, and right semitendinosis muscles. Though runs of high frequency discharges are seen, they are not neurotonic discharges. Their generalized nature and similar morphology in all channels (arrows) makes them more likely to be an artifact from an extraneous source.

ELECTROENCEPHALOGRAPHY

EEG monitoring is often used when vascular supply to the brain may be interrupted. Carotid endarterectomy (CEA) is a common indication for such monitoring. During CEA, if slowing is noted ipsilateral to the side of clamping of the carotid artery, bypass is considered. If slowing occurs, it is usually within a few minutes of clamping. Often, no change in the EEG is noted, implying adequate collateral perfusion.

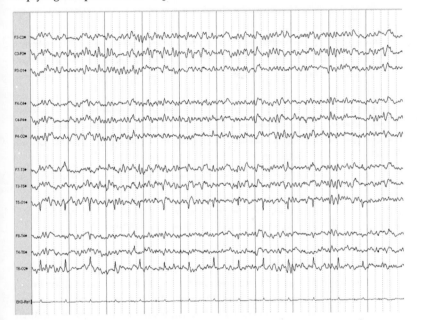

FIGURE 9.30. This is intraoperative EEG showing symmetric activity 3 minutes after clamping of the right carotid artery. The parameters of recording include a 30 mm/sec display speed, filter settings 1 to 70 Hz, and a sensitivity 7 μV/mm.

The patient shown above was undergoing a right CEA. This is a 10 second sample taken 3 minutes after clamping of the right carotid artery. The EEG continues to look symmetric implying adequate collateral circulation. Notice that Fp1 and Fp2 electrodes are absent; they were not applied because of presence of anesthesia probes in that location.

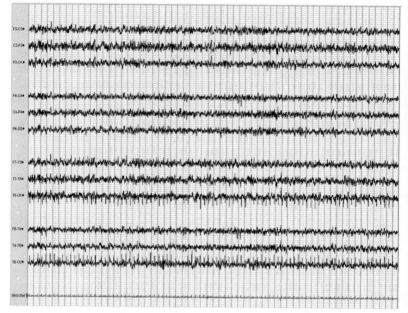

FIGURE 9.31. This is intraoperative EEG from the same patient as shown on the last page; this is 60 seconds of symmetric activity. The parameters of recording include a 15 mm/sec display speed, filter settings 1 to 70 Hz, and a sensitivity 7 µV/mm.

When monitoring EEG during CEA, often a 60 second page is useful as slowing and loss of faster frequencies are better visualized at slower paper speed. This sample is from the same patient and time as the last sample with a display of 60 seconds. The right carotid artery was clamped 3 minutes prior to this EEG. Notice the symmetry of both sides.

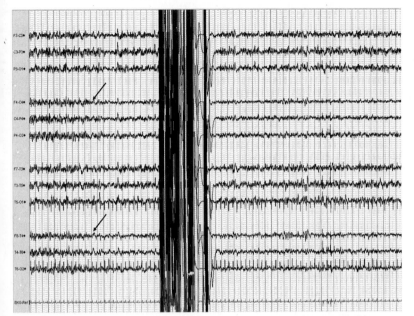

FIGURE 9.32. This is intraoperative EEG showing loss of faster frequencies over the right hemisphere after clamping of the right carotid artery. The parameters of recording include a 15 mm/sec display speed, filter settings 1 to 70 Hz, and a sensitivity 7 µV/mm.

As noted above, a slow paper speed can be helpful in identifying slow-ing and loss of faster frequencies. When slowing occurs, it is often within minutes of clamping the carotid artery and is used as an indication for using bypass. The patient shown above was undergoing a right CEA. Approximately one minute after clamping the right carotid there was loss of faster frequencies in that hemisphere (arrows). The clamp was removed, and the EEG returned to baseline. Notice that Fp1 and Fp2 electrodes are absent; they were not applied because of presence of anesthesia monitoring in that location.

CHAPTER 9

ADDITIONAL RESOURCES

James ML, Husain AM. Brainstem auditory evoked potential monitoring: when is change in wave V significant? *Neurology* 2005;65(10):1551-1555.

Journee HL, Polak HE, de Kleuver M, Langeloo DD, Postma AA. Improved neuro-monitoring during spinal surgery using double-train transcranial electrical stimulation. *Med Biol Eng Comput.* 2004;42:110-113.

Legatt AD. Mechanisms of intraoperative brainstem auditory evoked potential changes. *J Clin Neurophysiol.* 2002;19(5):396-408.

MacDonald DB. Safety of intraoperative transcranial electrical stimulation motor evoked potential monitoring. *J Clin Neurophysiol.* 2002;19(5):416-429.

Nuwer MR, Dawson EG, Carlson LG, Kanim LE, Sherman JE. Somatosensory evoked potential spinal cord monitoring reduces neurologic deficits after scoliosis surgery: results of a large multicenter survey. *Electroencephalogr Clin Neurophysiol.* 1995;96(1):6-11.

Radtke RA, Erwin CW, Wilkins RH. Intraoperative brainstem auditory evoked potentials: significant decrease in postoperative morbidity. *Neurology.* 1989; 39(2 Pt 1):187-191.

Robertson SC, Traynelis VC, Yamada TT. Identification of the sensorimotor cortex with SSEP phase reversal. In: Loftus CM, Traynelis VC. eds. *Intraoperative Monitoring Techniques in Neurosurgery.* New York: McGraw-Hill, Inc.; 1994:107-111.

Seyal M, Mull B. Mechanisms of signal change during intraoperative somatosensory evoked potential monitoring of the spinal cord. *J Clin Neurophysiol.* 2002;19(5):409-415.

Index

Index

*This book is dedicated to our families,
our fine colleagues interested in EEG,
our friends in the field of EEG technology,
and especially our patients.*

DKWILY